Weighting To Wait

The Emotions of Permanent Fat-Loss

Maximizing Your Latent
Emotional Strengths To Reach
Your Fat-loss Goals And
Sustain Them Once And For All.

by

Sovereign M. Valentine

http://sovereign-valentine.mykajabi.com

About The Author

Sovereign Valentine has invested the last two decades studying, experimenting and applying general fitness principles, as well as perfecting the principles contained herein.

After witnessing first-hand, the affects of poor lifestyle choices within his family and breaking free of the junk food and sugar addiction behaviors himself, he has been refining and practicing what he preaches for the last thirty years. During those decades, Sov personally invested tens of thousands of dollars over the years experimenting to find out what products and ideas are hoaxes and which ones are actually effective and work with everyone who commits to applying them.

Through an intensive and extensive trial-and-error process and by consistently doing what was purported to work he found what really *does* work. He then goes about documenting the results with each client.

In Sov's words, *"There is no longer a mystery to healthy, sustainable weight loss. The science and art have been figured out...there aren't any exceptions...it simply comes down to doing the correct things at the correct times and refining as you go. If you think you're an exception, you're not!"*

Sovereign began his formal training as a health care professional with a sincere desire to work with athletes. From a combination of formal training and decades of experimenting he developed a system that absolutely works.

Sovereign says, *"If you aren't burning between 12 and 20 pounds of fat per month, something is off. A properly designed and executed exercise and nutrition program will facilitate these numbers, (as well as improve overall health) unless you aren't following through correctly. Without a way to know if you're on track, weeks could go by and you wouldn't even know you're off track."*

In 1992 he became a Licensed Massage Therapist in Washington State. In 1994 he began doing small, informal nutrition presentations so that others could experience the profound impact that real nutrition has on the body. In 1996 he became a foot and hand reflexologist as well as an energetic healing master. In 1997 he became a certified hypno-therapist. In 1998 he began training others in hypnotherapy and in 1999 he became the first person ever at the school he attended to be certified as a Master Clinical Hypnotherapist. He went on to become certified in Fitness Training, Fitness Therapy, Sports Conditioning, Endurance Conditioning, a Specialist in Performance Nutrition as well as a Youth Conditioning Specialist, Golf Fitness Instructor, Senior Fitness Specialist, Community Emergency Response Team Member (CERT) and Licensed First-Responder.

Sovereign's thorough understanding of the systems of the body and how they relate to one another is reflected in his ability to fine-tune his clients' training and nutritional regimes for extra-ordinary *Results!*

His published works include *Reasons or Results Performance Nutrition Training, If I Were Her Trainer, Life-long Fat-loss System, Be Your Own Personal Trainer and 50-ish Reasons.*

Foreword

The weight loss industry as a whole has been evolving over the last hundred years, but especially so in the last forty years, as being overweight and obese, diabetes and all the other *dis*-eases that accompany being overweight have increased to epidemic proportions.

Generally speaking, the amount of information is simply crazy. But accurate, science-based information which produces healthy, consistent results, which can be maintained over the long-haul is simple in nature, but rare. Much of what's out there is simply about spewing marketing and advertising solutions for some problem symptoms (being overweight and in pain) and then saying, *"Here, take this and all your problems will be solved."*

The truth of the matter, after applying this kind of information for more than twenty years, on both myself and my clients, is that there truly are good nutritional products that make weight loss easier, faster and with less effort, but they are few and far between and the general public simply can't tell a good product from a ineffective one. That's a part of what I do...assure quality and success through health improvement to prevent and reduce suffering.

In the United States right now, the right people are doing the right research to help you get real *Results!* all the while 99% of food products and dietary supplements for sale really have little nutrition at all, resulting in a lot of missed opportunities by people who could have gotten better *Results!* but to this day don't know why they don't know.

When you hear the words "fad diet", what they're talking about is either a good program that people picked away at until there wasn't any relevant nutritional content left (requires lifestyle change). Or, the program promised weight loss, without exercise and nutritional density, to begin with. With any weight loss program, if the amount of nutritional density isn't increased and isn't provided to your body consistently, you simply won't stick with it, since there's no pay off to your chemistry of the brain and body, without additional, consistent nutrition density.

Secondly, any program that suggests you can burn off all the fat and gain health in all ways but is without some kind of resistance training [and] cardiovascular/aerobic exercise is a pipe dream designed to appeal to people who feel frustrated, depressed, sad, defeated and helpless...feeling like they can't do it anymore...empty promises...*hype*...-*a bait-and-switch.*

The true secret is finding a trainer who has your overall health in mind (not just short-term weight loss) [your health should be improving and you should be feeling better as time goes on] and a trainer who has enough expertise to not only design an amazingly effective program, but one who knows how to adjust the program to you for most effectiveness. Most trainers can design a program, but they don't know how to adjust the program if progress slows down or progress hits a plateau (accountability for both the client and the trainer). This is the second part of what I do.

One of the things that makes me so effective as a weight loss expert is that I've been doing this so long, that when a client isn't losing weight, I can narrow it down to whether it has something with the actual workouts, the thoughts & attitudes of the client, the nutritional aspect or if it's in the application of the program during the hours when the client isn't with me.

There simply aren't any mysteries to healthy, sustainable weight loss to me anymore. A majority of trainers don't stick with the industry long enough to find out what *they didn't know*...I have.

This book lays it out there in simple, concise, and states the basics from many angles and viewpoints, so there's no question what has to happen once you've completed this book.

When you apply these tactics in the way I show you here, you and those who know you will be blown away by the *Results!* you are getting. This book is for people who want the results that speak for themselves…anyone can lose weight...every "die-t" will produce some kind of results in the short-run, but most quick, weight loss programs erode the physical health after leaving you malnourished, tired, exhausted and depleted...resulting in gaining all the weight back and some additional weight.

Any health-building weight loss program should leave you feeling lighter, more clear, relaxed, rejuvenated and more vital than when you started, as well as free of all cravings and any attraction to junk food.

Apply this information and you will be so glad...*I promise.*

Read this book now; start getting better today and I look forward to seeing and hearing how good you feel about the *Results!* you are getting!

Once you've read the material, if you're the type to recognize what is real and not just the next fad and if you're willing to commit and follow through until the end, *I'll be there with you every step of the way.*

If this describes you, feel free to contact me for your complimentary consultation, as part of your purchase of this book.

Acknowledgments

I have not attempted to cite in the text all the authorities and sources in the preparation of this book. To do so would require more space than is available in order to effectively serve you who apply this information. The list would include departments of the federal government, libraries, industrial institutions, web sources and many individuals.

Inspiration was contributed by all those before me who succeeded as best they could with the information they had at the time, as well as all those after me who will improve upon this information to make the lives of others better. This book is a culmination of hundreds of books I've read, thousands of hours of experimentation and thousands of hours of observing the why, how and where of my own and others' successes and frustrated attempts.

A Word from the Author

Take everything you have already learned about weight loss and put it in a safe place (it does have a place and a purpose). BUT, what you thought you knew about the emotions in relation to weight loss and their accompanying nutritional principles may be preventing you from burning off all that fat once and for all. For what you're about to learn here is going to change your life forever and I can see how it will change the lives of those around you as well….in dramatic ways…for the better. By *applying* it! Just by doing it!

Now, not only will you get faster, more consistent *Results!,* you will also begin learning why you did *not* get results before. You will discover what was holding you back and interfering with your weight loss success before.

In order to lose weight and keep it off (body composition of 20% or less), the cells of your body, especially the brain must be consistently and fully fed. (Feeding the cells nutrition density is different from the action we know as eating). In other words, what you consume must get into the cells where they can make use of it. Taking supplements only helps if they make their way to your blood stream and your brain. The brain controls the emotions and the emotions determine when you follow through with your exercise and nutrition homework.

Weighting To Weight; The Emotions of Permanent Fat-Loss is an easy to follow outline for you to follow to get your body on track…better than ever.

At first, you will notice a marked difference, quite possibly without being able to say what that difference is. Then, as the days pass, you will notice a higher level of energy, and mental & emotional clarity like you've never had before coming to your exercise and nutrition habits. And it is at that point that you will realize that what you thought nutrition was about and what it really is are two different things.

This is a *do it* book…read it, learn it…*do it.* If you don't apply it as instructed, you'll miss out.

As I said in my first book, there are three major types of nutrition information out there now days: 1) theory-based nutrition on how things should be 2) medical-nutrition on how some medical professionals try to chase symptoms with nutrition and this book being 3) applied-nutrition.

Applied nutrition is a combination of three things that make for a no-miss, leave no stone unturned program: 1) whole-foods 2) functional-foods and 3) certain dietary supplements at certain times to fill in nutritional gaps everyone has.

Much of the information out there is a mixed bag of the three and that is part of the reasons people get such mixed and inconsistent results. If you are going to do this, then do it. Trust yourself enough to know you can do this stuff and monitor your experiences or ask me for help. But whatever you do, do not try to get someone from the other two categories to help you with *this* system…they simply will not understand it and you will likely quit before you get significant *Results!*.

The first 2-3 chapters are quite dense in that they discuss the foundation of bringing intangible emotional material to conscious awareness…don't be afraid to read those chapters a couple times before moving on!

Left to their own, emotional problems can become mental problems, *which become health problems.*

I will be happy to answer your questions about the material in this book. E-mail to set up your appointment for your personalized consultation.

If you're like me, the type of person who simply wants to be shown what to do, just ask! I have exactly what you need to succeed.

I work to make a living, but I live to see you get *Results!*

Sovereign Michael Valentine

March 2018.

Disclaimer

This book is designed to provide information about the subject matter covered. It is produced and sold with the understanding that the publisher and author are not engaged in rendering neither medical diagnosis nor treatment. If you need medical help, go get it. It is not the purpose of this manual to reprint all the information that is otherwise available from other health professionals but to complement, amplify and supplement other texts. *Weighting To Wait* is neither a cure-all nor a quick-fix for poor lifestyle habits or tendencies. Anyone who commits to personal accountability for their health must expect to re-direct some time, energy and money without any guarantee for specific benefits within a fixed time frame. *Nature works at her own pace.*

Every effort has been made to make this book as complete and accurate as possible. However, there may be mistakes both typographical and in content. Therefore, this book should be used as a general guide and not as the ultimate source of health and nutritional information. Your uniqueness will shine through as you succeed.

The purpose of this book is to educate and inform. The very best results will come from participation. Neither the publisher nor the author shall have responsibility to any person or entity with respect to any loss or damage caused by or alleged to be caused directly or indirectly by the information contained in this book. *The products referred to in this book carry their own satisfaction guarantee by the producer of the products and were not necessarily originally designed to be used in the order, context or manners described in this book.*

This book is not meant to replace the advice or treatments prescribed by your doctor, but rather to accompany your physician's advice. It is not meant to encourage medical treatment of illness or disease or any medical problem by the layperson. It is meant to inform you and open you to health choices that are available to those who seek a broader knowledge. Any application of the ideas set forth in this book is at the applicant's discretion and sole risk. If you are under a doctor's care for any condition, she or he can advise you *about information she or he is familiar with and which she or he has personally experienced.*

The information in this book is neither diagnostic nor prescriptive. It is informational only. The data and information contained herein are based upon information from various peer-reviewed, published and unpublished sources and merely represent training, experience, health and nutrition literature and practices summarized.

Neither the publisher nor the author of this book makes any warranties, expressed or implied regarding the currency, completeness or scientific accuracy or validity of this information nor does it warrant the fitness of the information for any particular purpose. It is intended to provide helpful and informative material on the subjects addressed in the publication. It is sold with the understanding that the publisher and author are not engaged in rendering medical, health, or any other kind of personal professional services in this book. The publisher and author specifically disclaim all responsibility for any liability, loss or risk, personal or otherwise which is incurred as a consequence, directly or indirectly, from the use and application of any of the contents of this book.

If you do not wish to be bound by the above terms, return this book to the place of purchase or to the publisher or author for a full refund of purchase price.

Table of Contents

Chapter One

What You Get From *Weighting To Wait*

What I'm going to show you within these pages is how to efficiently lose 12-20 pounds of fat *per month* in a health-building, safe, sustainable fashion and feel better than ever. What you'll have as results of this is freedom and more choices! Most successful models of behavioral change/improvement inherently enable a person to have more freedom and greater choice as to how you will live the rest of your life and this information will not disappoint.

In addition, you'll likely gain:

- More consistent and increased energy,

- Improved mental clarity,

- Greater emotional stability,

- Decreased cravings for unhealthy foods & beverages,

- Less frequent colds, flu & bugs,

- Relief from chronic health conditions,

- Improved sleep,

- Improved attention & concentration,

- A decrease in anxiety and nervousness,

- Greater clarity and perspective on your own life,

- Better, more properly responsive immune system and

- Dramatic improvement in motivation and consistency.

By freeing up yourself from the constant battle of weight gain/weight loss (and all the feelings and self-talk that go with that) you'll certainly have more time and freedom to do things, go places, meet people and all around have more fun! Isn't that a point of life anyway? To have more fun? Enjoy life more?

Your life will likely improve in many contexts by practicing and applying what you learn here, and you can look forward and expect to that. You can have faith that your future will be different now...*you can imagine this as a fresh start!*

Weighting To Wait unlocks one of the most important and critical factors that is also the single most overlooked and misunderstood principle of weight loss...*utilizing the emotions to fuel your success.*

By taking in the ideas in here and applying them, the mystery of weight loss will be revealed to you and you'll likely go on to help other with what has helped you...*paying it forward.*

You'll certainly be getting asked a lot of questions as to how you suddenly lost all the weight. Friends and family will want to know what finally made the difference for you.

In these pages I'm going to explain, show and tell you how to intervene on your own life, in order to take control of your health once and for all. Although the particular details here are about weight loss in general, you can apply these principles to all endeavors in all contexts of your life.

I'm going to explain to you how the misunderstandings and passive use of emotions, more or less sabotage one's ability to simply follow through on a given exercise and nutrition program...*simple misunderstandings.* Also, how to take charge once and for all by turning the table on emotions and get them working for you, rather than interfering and blocking your progress, so you can make get the consistent results you've been longing for.

By applying these principles, you'll likely have a few "light-bulb" moments..."a-ha" moments where you'll realize what has been happening just outside your awareness, so you can once and for all get-all-your-ducks-in-a-row, lining up your goals, intentions, motivation...*freeing you up to simply succeed.* Knowledge applied is power and you're now going to be in the driver's seat of your own weight loss journey. Personal power provides freedom.

As I was working my way through more nearly three decades experienceas, a personal trainer helping people from all walks of life achieve all sorts of fitness goals, (as well as reflecting on the dynamics of poor health and obesity in my own family), contrasting patterns began to emerge with the people who seemed to effortlessly reach their goals in contrast to the ones who struggled and often quit before they reached their goals, *regardless of which weight loss model they were participating in.*

I notice very clear behavioral distinctions between people who adhere to a fitness or weight loss program and the people who couldn't seem to get their mind in the game (for the sake of a clear distinction, imagine an Olympic athlete in contrast to a person who can't stop eating cake after their personal training session). The Olympic athlete can't afford the luxury of holding onto the past without it interfering in the present moment and future performance...*being present*. Or the Olympic athlete at least knows how to set 'feelings' aside long enough to successfully train and perform in their chosen event. Holding on to the past or the emotional aspect of the past (even if it's happening at an unconscious habit level) absolutely interferes in present moment, in fact it can prevent a person from being present at all.

Chapter conclusion:

By applying the strategies in here, you'll reach goals that you might have tried to reach numerous times before, but likely fell short. These concepts are likely the missing link to your continued and sustainable success...*now you have more choices!*

"You are an excellent trainer...you far exceeded my expectations...if anyone wants to know what you are like to train with have them call me personally and I'll tell them." J.DG., Seattle, WA

Chapter Two

The Evolution of Awareness

Although I began my professional career as a licensed massage practitioner in Washington State and evolving into a professional personal trainer, ultimately, every time I had a client whom had a condition I wasn't trained to help I would go get professional training in that particular modality. Even with all that education and training certifications, there was very little tangible material to rely on to recognize, map and address each clients' particular emotional paradigms, that were interfering in their progress to lose weight and keep it off.

There is obviously an emotional component with every person who wants and needs to lose weight, but without a big picture model that in some ways applies to every person, you effectively have to learn every person's way of dealing with emotions, every single time (meaning create a new model for every person)...which is simply too time consuming to help people in a reasonable time frame for them to stay motivated and overcome previous stumbling stones. What I found is that the "context" or structure of emotional issues is the same for everyone (for some reason, people can have clear goals but if their trainers isn't right there with them 24/7, walking them through their feelings as they experience them, they regress back to the emotions which got them over weight to begin with...as though the emotional state has such a grasp on their intellect that they can't see outside of it long enough to adhere to their weight loss program). There's 168 hours in a week and most clients spend only three or less hours with their trainer each week, at best.

Once I had realized, mapped and cross-referenced the emotional pattern commonalities (the big picture/commonalties/common denominators) [the outward manifestations of emotions] with all clients who seemed "stuck", the intangible aspect of emotional interruption became very tangible and clear...I could see and hear exactly what was interfering with the clients' mind, as it was happening...even when *they* weren't conscious of it happening....they could feel the feelings associated, but couldn't get a "meta" or 'perspective from above' (also known as having an experience, but having perspective on the experience at the same time/sentience) on what they were experiencing enough to get a handle on it, change it and prevent it from interfering in their progress. And even when a client is verbally "encoding" what the real problems were (encoding meaning: *having an experience but calling it something else to avoid the feelings associated with it*) they aren't able to have enough self-awareness to *interrupt* the processes.

In other words, since the emotional problems were often rooted in emotional pain and subsequently suppressed (pushed down/disassociated), to some degree or another the client wouldn't say exactly what was bothering them or getting in their way, but might say something like, *"I walked past a bakery last night and saw a cake...I took it home and was going to eat a piece, but then ate the whole cake...I feel so bad."* And this would come from a client who just plunked down a lot of money for a personal training package. In other words, even if they had been through a ton of therapy, they might say the symptom of eating cake but be unable to verbalize the underlying problem that drive/enable eating the cake.

The common denominator, or how to 'know'/recognize the emotional drama, is [any behavior that is not in alignment with the prescribed exercise and nutrition program the client has agreed to].

At this point in the conversation with the client, the details (eating cake) become irrelevant since the unspoken content is the driver behind unconscious sabotage (even though the details might "seem" important from a personal training standpoint) (meaning the cake is just the outward symptom of the inside emotions)...with emotional interference, the details don't matter as much as noticing what's occurring (having feelings which are so overwhelming that they drive/control your behaviors without being able to stop the behaviors you don't want to experience, even when they are in conflict with what your stated goals are).... *"I can't eat just one, but I want to lose weight".*

Fitness industry weaknesses:

Unfortunately, a lot of personal trainers get into the industry hoping to get rich quick, earn a high hourly rate only to find that it takes a while to build up a consistent, motivated, appreciative clientele. Also unfortunate is the fact that the majority of trainers don't stick with the industry long enough to figure out what things they were telling their clients that were *incorrect,* how to design really *effective* exercise & nutrition programs and more importantly how to *adjust* the program when a program isn't effective for particular clients. This phenomenon tends to leave a trail of people who have "tried" to lose weight, even going as far as hiring a personal trainer, but then not quite making it or being abandoned by their trainer who was frustrated in their seemingly inability to affect change in the client. *Loving fitness isn't enough to help others escape their own downward spiral of emotional suppression.*

I would guess that few, if any, personal trainer certification courses cover the emotional aspects of weight loss and never have a I seen anything that comes close to the principles herein. Even some advanced programs don't cover the emotions of weight loss in ways that effectively help people get much faster results than they ever have before. Most personal training is effective with people who don't have emotional interference going on...these are the people who simply show up for their workouts and simply do the workouts and stick to their nutrition program without interference, from emotional fluctuations...*hint, hint.* For the most part, if someone is stuck in their emotions they're thought of as needy, neurotic or mentally ill, since you can't seem to get through to them...regardless of what or how many professional letters are behind the trainer's name and regardless of how many hours the trainer puts into explaining exercise and nutrition...after all, it took me thirty years to get here and I have more education, experience and broader learning base than a lot of personal trainers.

What compounds the problem further is if you get a personal trainer who doesn't even understand their own emotional personality...*you can't give what you don't have.*

But, I will tell you that those who apply this will likely get such great clarity of their previous struggles that there won't be any need to have the troubles any more.

In my experience, I learned the most from my clients who had clear goals during their initial intake, whom couldn't seem to simply follow through with proven exercise and nutrition programs that always work as long as they are followed through on, had some kind of emotional interference going on, in the background. These lessons were hard-won, since the information I needed most didn't seem to be available. We know the science of exercise and nutrition, it simply works when you apply it. Lack of emotional clarity seems to be the single greatest inhibitor of good intentions.

What doesn't work is trying to do exercise and nutrition while ignoring or talking "around" or "about" emotions. Acknowledging emotions exist isn't an antidote to emotional interference, since it doesn't address the reasons for the emotions interfering with exercise. Usually what a client says the emotional problem is, is only the very surface with the real content being suppressed underneath, often outside their awareness. Like the tip of an iceberg, healthy emotional balance means being able to experience emotions to enhance life, but being meta to them so they don't take over and run the show, no become your identity...*emotions are best suited for enhancing life experiences versus being the overbearing locus of life,* but people who are stuck in their emotions will adamantly dispute this point...effectively pointing out that emotions are the problem (...thou protest too much!).

More often than not, clients who have this emotional dichotomy going on think that once they say they have emotional stuff going on they have a hall-pass to skip workouts and binge on junk food. That's how you know they talked "around" the real issues but didn't release the issues. It's not the goal or intention to force a person to emote, but rather notice what they're experiencing, let them know it's healthy to feel the emotions, intently name them, then continue to feel them as they keep doing the actions of exercise and nutrition. Another hint for trainers, is that if the client insists they can't move forward, it's another likely indicator of emotional interference. Emotions often cuase a feeling of paralysis...the solution for which are the three parst fo nutrition combined with activity/motion (exercise structured to burn fat).

People who tend to be stuck in life are essentially and unwittingly tapping into the emotional part of life exclusively, to the point where they can't navigate other ways of "being"...*like being stuck in a rut without awareness that there is a whole world outside the rut.* People who do lead a healthy, lean life and find it effortless to do their nutrition and exercise aren't allowing themselves to get stuck in emotional based rut...*simply two sides of the same coin.* The people who are stuck in an emotional rut tend to say, *"Yay, but, what I feel is..."* whereas a person who isn't stuck might say, *"Yay, what I think is..."* In other words, even the language the emotionally stuck person uses often reflects what is going on inside their mental-emotional mind...*being overly focused on "feelings" as a crutch* to prevent forward movement...the safe feeling of staying stuck is in keeping the "feelings" pressed down instead of simply letting them go. The person who is stuck in their feelings (over-using/over reliance on their emotions) can't utilize their rational mind consistently enough to think their way out of problem that is emotionally-based...the strategy of the habit that started as a coping mechanism doesn't work to solve the problem, nor access a more productive state. Ultimately, if this dynamic isn't recognized and addressed, the client will adapt by using the emotions as a scapegoat to not do their workouts and binge on junk food. This is very common.

Regardless of which model a person uses to cope with life, they learned how to do their model at some point, became so good at it that they forgot they chose to do it in the first place and then do more and more of what isn't working without knowing they have created such a habit. The idea of 'sentience' or a 'sentient being' is that humans are supposed to be able to have thoughts, but think about their thoughts *as they are having them.* If you can't think about your thoughts, as you're having them, you aren't very likely to have control over your behaviors and often in direct conflict with your stated outcomes (weight loss/being healthy).

What is it that people are talking about, but not saying?

In wracking my brain, as to the specifics of why people who insist they want to lose weight can't even stick with a program they shelled thousands of dollars out for, outside the training sessions (whether it was hourly sessions or prepaid monthly packages), answers began to come. After that I could see where those answers fit the clients who had the most difficult time reaching their goals and inability in sustaining the results they got.

As a trainer or person on your own weight loss quest, once you get "it", you'll see how it's happening around you also. It's one of those things that once you're really aware of it, you can't ignore it. The key being that you have to make the corrections in yourself, before you can help others with it...a reason being that if your emotions aren't clear, your emotions and others' emotions kind of overlap and get all mixed up where you can't tell what's yours and what's theirs (e.g. two people who lack emotional clarity, being triggered off each other). One place to start is to notice where you insist you have to do something or can't stop yourself from doing something...*and then question it.* For example, skipping a workout or skipping your B.N.B.B.s.

Another Catch-22, in that regard is that people tend to migrate toward and hang out with people at a similar level of mental-emotional development. So, one way to look at it is that your mental-emotional equivalency will be an average of the five people you're around the most (more on this when we talk relationships). In other words, if you hang out with a group of people who all struggle with sticking to a plan and getting and staying lean, what do you think your average mental-emotional states will be? How likely are you to reach your goals if your circle of influence enables you to stay stuck: *"We love you just how you are.".*

The lesson here is that *some* people strive to raise their mental-emotional state to match their goals and do so by picking their circle of influence...athletic, healthy, fit-types especially. While people who avoid letting things go and moving on will often surround themselves with people who inadvertently enable them to stay within the comfort zone and keep the emotions suppressed and *dis*-associate from the knowledge of the habit itself. That doesn't mean giving up all your friends. It does point to increasing your circle of influence to at least include some people who are associated in the present time, have experience whether considered good or bad and then learning the lesson and moving on to the next step in life. An extreme example of this, would be addicts hanging out with other addicts. The comfort comes in being "enabled" to keep doing the habits which are not in your best interest, as we can always find people to love and accept us whether we are treating ourselves healthy or not. The addict mind will say they hang with people who accept them and love them for who they are, but we know this to be enabling and co-dependent behavior that sabotages one's ability to carry out goals, that are in conflict with the groups' mental-emotional mentality.

So, yes, I am saying a main factor that prevents people from losing weight once and for all is lack of clarity and misunderstandings about their emotions...they are effectively "having" emotions (indulging in unproductive states) (allowing unproductive emotions to inhabit their mind/body)...experiencing them, but not benefiting from them nor are the emotions adding any quality their life the way they could.

When people are run by their underlying emotions, suppress their emotions, deny what they are really feeling and call their feelings something other than what they are, they often feel out of control, seem to lack self-control, seem to lack conviction and integrity, and can't seem to follow through, as well as make decisions that conflict with what they say their goals are. A possible reason being that they don't feel they can express their true self, so they substitute with expression of "emotionally safe" ideas which are not personal to them. When people are being run by their emotions, they tend to be moved to say things and do behaviors that are not in their best interests. I'll cover some of the why's of this later.

But, when people realize their emotions are meant to be experienced and released they begin to have *"aha"* moments. In other words, the feeling of being overwhelmed begins to unwind and they begin having emotional stability and rational thought which aligns with their goals and intentions. If this describes you and you begin to get how to let stuff go, people who know you will make comments that you look younger and lighter (suppressed emotions make people look older than they are). When people stop pressing down the emotions, the behaviors that are a match for their goals become effortless (exercise & nutrition)...there's no interference and they tend to describe a feeling of "...*a weight being lifted,*" and knowledge that "...*it was never their job..,*" to be carrying that much emotional weight on their shoulders nor their responsibility of carrying the "weight" for everyone else, which shows up as excess body-fat, depression, anxiety and all the symptoms that go with it (lack of energy & motivation, high blood sugar, high blood pressure, sore joints, high cholesterol, etc.).

So, what I want you to get here is the contrast between [being run around by emotions] that seem to have a mind of their own versus [utilizing emotions as fuel/drivers toward your goals].

In my experience, more often than not, people who have difficulty adhering to their weight loss plan are simply being driven by emotions which have had free reign...emotions that are from the past, yet haven't been released or turned over.

Emotions are what we utilize to drive ourselves and motivate ourselves toward what we most want, but that only happens when people "utilize" their emotions versus the emotions "using" them to express what has been suppressed.

In other words, it's as though an unspoken rule of nature that [expression] is a higher priority to overall health than the behaviors of exercise and fitness...the body has to clear itself emotionally, first and foremost. What this tells is that one original driver of excess weight gain is unexpressed/suppressed/contained emotions.

Exercise and nutrition are part of three priorities, but without emotional clarity, no amount of exercise and nutrition can override the catastrophic effects of suppressed emotions. Again, the details/content/personal stories (content) don't count so much as the idea of suppression in general and where interference is occurring (context). The people who seem to easily work out and eat healthy have more efficient habits for dealing with stress and disappointments...and their strategies can be modeled, copied, taught and learned simply by hanging out around them...as long as you aren't trying to refine your own unhealthy coping habits by taking what they do and changing it to continue a suppression strategy.

In other words, you have to be willing to change the way you interact with the world, and how you react to the world to match your new goals versus trying to continue suppressing. In more technical terms, emotions (*in*tangible things) affect the physical being (tangible) by way of information transduction (changing ideas into chemical messengers) and by affecting the autonomic nervous system and vagus nerve via thoughts effecting the physical body.

What permits the emotions to be/stay suppressed?

Once this phenomena of emotional interference is recognized, the next most important question is what keeps the emotions suppressed? What permits it? What allows the emotions to stay suppressed versus being *expressed*? (especially when a person wants to lose weight). If its healthier to express than suppress, what permits suppression (this will be covered more fully in relation to the B.N.B.B.s and higher-level functioning of the brain, specifically nutrition density/types of calories), but for the time being...Also, holding the breathe enables stress and emtions to remain suppressed, which exercise reverses.

What wouldn't one just express?

Then the next question became why wouldn't one just express them? Just let them go? (related to what habit a person has learned or developed in coping with stress and disappointment before they knew they were learning).

Again patterns emerged: The clients who are (in the initial stages of weight loss; *e.g. first three months of a program*) beginning to express or let go of the suppressed emotions generally feel like they are paralyzed by the emotions, even though the emotions that are coming up, are not from things happening in the moment...the suppressed emotions are from incidents from times past but which were not dealt with at the time they occurred (the times when the client suppressed the experience rather than experiencing it and letting it go). Again, the details/content/story don't matter. If a person is too attached to the details of their story, they may mistake telling the story over and over instead of releasing it (affiring it instead of relaeasing it)...they identify with it too much, and instead of letting it go and moving forward, they hold onto it like a possession and keep telling the same story, but are not growing/evolving/improving as a person. Retelling the story makes it a driver of your identity, as opposed to having an experience.

Remember, emotions are meant to be experienced (to enhance life) and then released. Any emotions that are bottled up ultimately are going to strive to surface...but as they do, the person experiencing them generally doesn't realize that the feelings they are having are the old emotions *LEAVING* their body...but emotions feel the same whether they are first occurring, or being suppressed and then kept down as they do when they are finally be released. The struggle or intensity of the emotions [is from trying to keep them suppressed] versus simply feeling them, acknowledging them and setting them free. All the "feelings" are the *struggle* or difficulty of holding the feelings in instead of just letting them go...*kind of a struggle between what feel snormal and what is healthier.* Along with that is keeping them in but keeping them just outside awareness so they are influencing the self but not understanding how or why.

Break through:

A key to making progress and consistent, long-term success is learning to be present enough to know if what you are feeling is from recycling the past (depression), being present in the moment (excitement & motivation) or anticipating the future (anxiety).

Where does the energy to keep suppressing come from?

So, considering how much energy it takes to keep emotions bottled up, how could someone constantly have enough energy to keep them like that?

S.A.D.C.R.A.P. calories...(usually nutrition-deficient calories). Calories are the metabolic equivalent of a boat anchor...the more calories a person consumes the more emotion they can suppress and the bigger the container they make (body-fat)...but the bigger the container they make, the more emotions they suppress and the more calories they have to consume to keep the new level of emotions suppressed...the endless cycle we know as yo-yo dieting....*Weighting To Wait.* Exercise reduces the size of the container, so the emotions move on, are released or "come out of the body".

A paradox here is that nutritionally-empty foods provide the caloric fuel to suppress emotional content, but in order to release and cope in a healthy way with life's stressors, a high amount of nutritional-density is consistently required.

This phenomena is related to which types of calories are consumed, which parts of the brain benefit from the different kinds of calories (nutritionally deficient, refined sugars, salt, bad fats and caffiene vs nutritionally dense whole-foods, functional-foods and supplemental B.N.B.B.s), how the energy is being used by the brain and which parts of the brain are being used to make decisions and physically feed the body (depending what part of the brain is primarily responsible for the hands choosing foods at any given time)[the well-nourished brain causes the hands to grab nutritionally-dense things, while the malnourished brain causes the hands to grab nutritionally-deficient things). The higher functioning parts of the brain require nutrition density, which is the opposite of suppressing emotions. The ability to carry out goals is the result of the higher functioning/frontal brain having adequate B.N.B.B.s.

In essence, the person suppressing the emotions is waiting to find a way to get rid of the feelings without feeling them (unnatural). The net result of "waiting" for the feelings to go away on their own is adding "weight" to their body! *...also known as "weighting".* Emotions have to be felt and then let go!

How this plays out in real time is someone gets a personal training session, and after their workout (being influenced by old emotions surfacing during the workout), they skip the B.N.B.B.s (Basic Nutritional Building Blocks) and nutrition in general, see a cake in the bakery window telling themselves they'll just have a taste and then since they are so deficient of the B.N.B.B.s they eat the whole cake...then the cycle starts over...afterward they often have strong feelings of guilt and shame about eating the whole cake but instead of letting those feelings go and getting on track, they suppress the feelings with more calories required to meet the energy required to keep the new batch of emotions suppressed, on top of all the previous emotions. Then the person feels so bad they disassociate (distance themselves emotionally from themselves) from their behaviors. So, for all intent and purpose they have no "presence of mind" about what they have done. To relieve themselves of the behavior they allowed to go on, they "check out" from the experience which reinforces the behavior into a more ingrained, unconscious habit. The side effect is weight gain/high body-fat.

Shocking!

What causes a person to start an exercise program, but not follow through? Usually, there is some incident (like seeing a candid picture of themselves) which temporarily shocks them into present time (being associated) when they go ask a trainer for help or join a weight loss group saying they need help and something to the effect of, *"One day I woke up and I was fat...I don't recognize myself"* (indicating they weren't present in their body/disassociated (living a distance from themselves) enough to the affects they were having on their physical being) [too absorbed in emotional experiences running in the background].

Once some time has passed (about three months) they are distant enough from the shock of really seeing themselves, they give themselves permission (because they have done "such a good job") for some more food that disassociates them from present time, they start missing workouts and the process starts over…*partly because of the familiarity of S.A.D.C.R.A.P. feels good to the undernousihed brain (lack of B.N.B.B.s)*.

Most of the time, a person living with these dynamics will, during the initial intake, tell the trainer or weight loss coach about their lack of exercise, what they are eating, but very little of what the emotional drivers are, since they are literally unaware of what strategy they have been doing to get where they are. Often there was a misunderstanding in their mind before they were old enough to make critical decisions, but intended to get relief from a stressor...they did the best they could with what they had at the time.

After more than thirty years of working with people professionally, I'm convinced that simply getting associated and being present within the mind and body triggers the response needed to start the process of getting lean and healthy, but maintaining the state takes extra nutritional support. The outcome for the trainer of health care provider is to replace the *dis*-associative states with habits and lifestyle improvement which trigger the state of being present, even when their trainer isn't present..*anchor the feeling*/help make it permanent. Like any addiction to comfort there's always the temptation to take the easy route and just not do the behaviors that will get you what you say you want...as long as *dis*-association is occurring, it's just easier not to.

But emotions are not physical things!

Body-fat is the equivalent of a dynamic, virtual storage container. Much of the fitness industry perceives body-fat as a symptom of eating too much and too little activity. In reality, body-fat and all the accompanying physiological side effects are the outward symptoms of the psyche needing more room to contain an ever-increasing amount of suppressed emotional content...a virtual, emotional storage barrel.

A major paradox is that even if the amount of emotional-content does not increase, since nature wants the emotions to be released and the person to move on with life, it takes increasingly more and more nutrient-lacking calories to keep the *same* amount of emotional-content suppressed. The Catch-22 is that most people don't stop there, they unconsciously and habitually pile on more and more emotional-content attempting to cover the initial content more deeply, where hopefully it stays beyond conscious awareness...this is because the process works more efficiently as time goes on, to make the person feel better than the first few times they did it.

In fact, the concept of "perfecting a neurosis" where a person has stuffed emotions away, has symptoms (often inconsistent, un-diagnosable symptoms that change as fast as they are noticed, *e.g. pain, discomfort, anxiety, depression, etc.*), for which they go to a doctor, nurse, physician assistant or trainer or whomever they choose only to refute that they need to exercise and improve their nutritional habits.

You see, unconsciously they know what the problem is and refuse to do the exercise and nutrition. So, in a cry for help seek professional guidance to keep doing what they are doing but get the results of people who eat better and exercise consistently...."perfecting the neurosis", e.g. *"I want to lose weight but I can't exercise or stop eating S.A.D.C.R.A.P."* ..."Please give me the pill that will allow me to keep suppressing my feelings but lose weight anyway!"..."I want to lose weight, but this pain won't allow me to exercise...I need people to do my stuff for me!"*

Known solutions:

The most direct way I have seen to interrupt this cycle is to 1) Reduce the [nutrient deficient] calories while simultaneously 2) Increasing [nutrient density in the daily routine/the B.N.B.B.s] which enables being present in the moment, versus foods that enable *dis-association* (S.A.D.C.R.A.P.) and do the activities (properly designed fat-burning exercises) to burn the fat. The results being that the virtual emotional container shrinks (fat-loss) and the suppression affect reverses. In other words, the excessive body-fat and accompanying emotions are the classic paradox of, *"What came first, the chicken or the egg?".* Did you start suppressing emotions and gain fat to contain them or did you gain fat to hold the emotions in? Either way, the solution is the same...*strategic activity and increased nutrition density.*

Without adequate, daily nutrition density on board in the brain, the person simply won't feel mentally/emotionally prepared to cope with and let go the emotional-content they had been suppressing...they get stuck in the phase of emotional pain and can't seem to move through it. When people have enough nutritional content on board, in the higher functioning areas of their brain, they simply experience the emotional-content and *let it go*...they don't get stuck. Historically, there have been counselors and therapists who find that without adequate nutrition in the brain, patients simply can't move forward, since the function of the brain follows chemistry, which is built from the B.N.B.B.s.

Whether it's a couple who can't get along or prisoners or troubled youth, their ability to cope and exercise emotional stability, nutrition density is key. A reason being that it takes immense mental capacity to process cognitive material and the pre-frontal cortex (front of the brain) has to be fueled in order to do so, otherwise people can't get past the emotional pain they are experiencing...[being in pain is not enough of a motivation to be able to process cognitive material]...unfortunately, the pre-frontal cortex seems to be the last part of the brain to get enough nutrition, since it is an area that is responsible for rational thought, recognition of love and compassion and being able to think your way out of emotional challenges. Rational though requires nutrition!

Since the pre-frontal cortex isn't responsible for functions of the body per se, (like the heartbeat), nutritional resources aren't distributed there until all the other areas get their share. The brain prioritizes gaining pure energy (glucose/sugar/junk food/S.A.D.C.R.A.P.) over nutrition density and when you combine a high stress(ors) followed by nutrition that is inadequate for the situation, the net results are an emotional pain, suppression, binge-continuous cycles that can't effectively be escaped /eliminated without intervening with higher than average amounts of nutrition density (B.N.B.B.s).

Ultimately, what I have found is that in some ways, people are set up to either be a person who has an experience and let's it go or a person who experiences something and suppresses the emotions down inside the body (each persn's constitution). Some people learn healthy coping skills early while others learn suppression early in life.

The Olympic athlete for example doesn't afford themselves the luxury, the indulgence of holding on to the past or suppressing emotions down, since this literally interferes with their ability to physically perform. One person is choosing to let go the past in exchange for what's ahead, while the overweight/obese person places higher value (albeit unconsciously to an extent) on controlling feelings, pressing the past down and then having to consume greater and greater calories to have the energy to do so and thereby creating a bigger and more dense container to hold more and more emotional-content (in order to feel safe, from the inside-out). The greatest components for emotional suppression are what I refer to as S.A.D.C.R.A.P. (Standard American Diet of Continuously & Repetitively Advertised Products)...*the most commonly advertised junk food.* I refer to them as this because my clients tell me they think, *"... they feel sad and look like crap...,"* after they consume it, even when they initially are convinced they couldn't do without it.

S.A.D.C.R.A.P. is a double-edged sword because it contains the 'caloric energy' to suppress emotional pain, but the chemical content and artificial ingredients are a chemical concoction which create a *dis-*associated state like alcohol or any other addictive substance...feel-good chemicals and substances that "feel good" while they are affecting the brain, but leave the brain even more depleted and malnourished (Catch-22)...permitting some people to suppress and then through state-dependent behavior, forget the extent they suppressed after the fact...every time they start to feel the content surfacing, they take another serving of S.A.D.C.R.A.P. and the cycle is reinforced.

Without adding significant nutrition density, e.g. 1) Whole-foods 2) Functional-foods and 3) Certain dietary supplements at certain times, you effectively allow the suppression to continue.

Without adding in the nutritional density which enables the person to process the emotional material with their pre-frontal cortex/upper brain, they have effectively been left vulnerable to the withdrawl symptoms of S.A.D.C.R.A.P. When you have enough B.N.B.B.s on board, you don't experience any cravings. Cravings are side effects of not enough nutrition in the brain, for your situation. Cravings are side effects of not enough nutrition, for your situation.

A *part* of depressed feelings people experience is that they are so focused on the past there's no emotional energy left to fully enjoy the present (exercise and eating healthier). Secondly, so much energy being used to suppress emotions they don't have energy left to enjoy the present. (It's very common for people experiencing this phenomena to deny it...they haven't made the decision to change and they are in fear that if they do begin feeling, it will just be more negativity...they can't see the light at the end of the tunnel).

The next level of progress comes when the person begins eating more healthy and doing activities that begin to reduce the overall mass of the a dynamic, virtual storage, containment system known as body-fat. As a person improves the nutritional status of their brain, the functioning of the brain moves from primarily emotional *to cognitive and rational.* Once the brain is functioning more cognitively the person is able to tell the difference between emotional feeling-based-thoughts and cognitive rational-based-thoughts, they generally realize they were being manipulated by their emotions and their thoughts and behaviors were tainted by emotions.

As the dynamic, virtual storage, containment system known as body-fat begins reducing in size and mass, the emotional-content doesn't have as much area to inhabit and the content (e.g. the details, the stories, the feelings) may begin to surface into conscious awareness, not unlike flashbacks that veterans with PTSD experience. As the content surfaces, the person may have physical sensations as well.

One of the dichotomies of this process though is that people who generally suppress emotions rather than simply experience them and let them go is that as the emotions begin to leave the body, the details of what were related to those emotions also surface into consciousness, although [it doesn't have to/isn't required]. In other words, for lack of better terms, the person is experiencing present time experience as well as the content of the emotions from long ago. This duality of emotional experience can be overwhelming for many people. In a different context, there's a paradoxical saying that, *"...dying is easy, it's the trying to be alive and not be in pain that's hard".*

In relation to weight loss (fat-loss), it actually uses more physical energy (calories) to keep emotions suppressed than it is to simply let the content go…notice that people who are fit and healthy often eat less, appear smaller, yet have more physical and mental energy! But, for people who haven't developed the coping skills to simply let the emotional-content go, nor consumed enough nutritional density to trigger cognitive-motivated functioning versus emotional-motivated functioning, it seems easier to keep doing what they are used to doing. The idea of experiencing the details of past events as it leaves the body can seem overwhelming (it's simply having feelings). If you've ever watched the television show *The Biggest Loser,* where in the first days of training the contestants begin to feel being alive they insist they can't even walk on a treadmill...they throw themselves down, have temper tantrums, scream, puke, pass out and so on....the feelings seem so real, they are convinced they can't move forward (they are simply having feelings and holding onto them), essentially a tantrum.

Without being on a show at a camp you can't leave, with cameras and trainers and so on, these behaviors just manifest as skipping a workout(s) and consuming S.A.D.C.R.A.P. and repeating the suppression cycle.

People who tend to have experiences, take the lesson and let the emotions go tend to seem light-hearted and positive, whereas as people who tend to hold onto or suppress emotions, tend to put keeping the feelings at bay and make a higher priority holding onto hurts, resentments and past pains and have a heavier emotionality to their personality...often relying on prescriptions in attempt to cover up their feelings of heaviness and anxiety even more artificially. The people who tend to let go of emotions tend to move forward quickly, simply doing what has to be done to reach their goals, versus behaving as though life is moving too quickly and behaving as if they have to stop or slow life down to accommodate them...*pointing to events that weren't processed fully at the time they happened (lack of integration).* There are cases where people have to have prescription medication, but that's beyond the scope of this book and between you and your doctor.

The point being that suppressing emotions takes so much of the life force or daily allotment of energy that the person who has excess body-fat cannot split their focus too far away from suppressing without the emotional-content simultaneously beginning to release from their hold within the body-fat, and then moving through consciousness and out of the body for good. Ultimately, we learn these patterns from those we're around the most as children, but sometimes it develops independent of others, especially if neglect was involved. As an adult, where it came from isn't as important as acknowledging the process and taking responsibility for it.

Commonalities among the two different groups (people who simply let it go and move on versus people who "contain" painful experiences), is that they expanded on whatever coping mechanisms they are using before they knew they were learning them! In other words, we mostly learn a model of dealing with emotions and experiences from our immediate environment before we even are mature enough to know we are learning. What that dynamic does is enable a person or empower them to copy how their family deals with emotions and if they go outside how their family deals with emotions there may be subtle consequences for doing things differently than the rest of the family. At the same time, once you know this it's up to you to *acknowledge it, become aware of it and change it.*

There are some people who are the only fat person in their family and what this sometimes reflects is that the family model of dealing with emotions wasn't a close enough fit for them, so they had a misunderstanding at a very young age and the person made a decision at some level, often before they can conceive the full implications of their decision and how their particular coping mechanisms would impact their health and body-fat level later in life.

I have seen the phenomena where one person in the family seems to take on the responsibility of "containing emotions" or "carrying" for the whole family and they end up as the only member who has excessive body-fat and everyone "wonders" why.

The whole concept of "comfort-food" points to this phenomena...when someone feels uncomfortable with what they are "feeling" and the feelings begin to surface into consciousness where one would otherwise use their coping skills to experience it and simply let it go, they rely on calorie dense (albeit absent of nutrition density) food & drink to suppress the discomfort back down into the body. Yes, S.A.D.C.R.A.P. enables suppression and *dis*-association via lack of nutritional density to the brain and by introducing chemicals into the brain which disable higher level, cognitive functioning of the pre-frontal cortex and by stimulating the emotional areas of the brain (limbic area), which triggers choices based on emotions versus rationale..."feelings" prioritized over thinking.

With each dose of emotional-content that gets suppressed, the container (body-fat) has to get bigger and denser to continue doing the function of containing the fat.

In case you didn't get it by now, properly executed exercise and nutrition density are the antithesis of being fat...*they can't co-exist*. You could have a person who considers themselves "active", insists they exercise all the time, insists they eat right and still be fat, but regardless of what the person thinks of their activity level, activity that burns fat is specific, not random movement in general (it involves calculating your resting heart rate, body composition and caloric requirements the first of each month). Additionally, if the body and brain (especially the brain) doesn't have enough nutrition density, no amount of activity will deliver permanent results, since the body also requires nutrition density (Basic Nutritional Building Blocks/B.N.B.B.s) to open up the energy pathways so that the body uses fat for energy and preserves the carbohydrate and protein for lean mass (muscle, bone density, organs, tissues...everything except body-fat). Third, as described earlier, without fueling and nourishing the higher functioning areas of the brain, most people won't successfully process emotional content/details, since doing so is a higher function of the brain, which requires adequate B.N.B.B.s for you.

Until the individual takes responsibility for this ongoing drama, they will insist they want to lose weight, even plunk down the big bucks for personal training and medical evaluation(s), but then insist that no matter what any expert they hire says, insist it doesn't apply to them and that no one understands them (the suppressed emotions talking) instead of the higher functions of the cognitive brain. That's one way to check yourself and increase your own presence of mind...What responses do you have?...What do you say and how do you respond when you receive information about nutrition? Truth be told, it's not others' responsibilities to understand what you experienced, its unique to you. It does feel better when others can understand us, so we don't feel so alone, but using others' lack of understanding to rationalize lack of follow through isn't fair to you or them!

When the bottom line is that you are habitually suppressing and asking others to diagnose outward signs and symptoms to a problem most people don't even know about and you haven't been able to speak about, you can go to a hundred practitioners, but they aren't going to be able to help you with something you aren't being honest with yourself about. The twist is that as long as you aren't present in your body and mind, you'll insist, *"... no one understands me,"* and that they don't have the answers...the answers are inside you and you have to let them out!...while you're exercising and getting adequate nutrition.

Chapter conclusion:

We know that properly designed exercise and nutrition programs work! Now we know that what often prevents people from simply doing the exercise and nutrition is inner, emotional-conflict. Once you learn to manage your emotions, rather than letting your emotions run you, weight loss is easy and sustainable. Left to their own, without intervention, imbalanced emotions can become influencers of the mental capacity and the mental capacity can affect overall quality of health outcomes. Meaning, if you don't manage your emotions, when you have the chance, the emotions affect physological processes and those affect physical health/weight/body composition through information-transduction (the brain taking ideas and converting them into brain chemicals/neuro-transmitters), which in-turn control behaviors: The well-nourished brain craves healthy, whole-foods and has the hands grab heathier choices. The under-nourished brain craves SADCRAP, makes choices based on immediate, emotional-satisfaction and has the hands grab SADCRAP, thereby sabotaging consistency in weight loss efforts.

No single, greater factor influences and helps assure weight loss success than consistent, correct application of the B.N.B.B.s, *without substitution.* How I know a client won't succced is when they insist they want my help, but also insist on changing the program. In these cases, I refer them to someone else.

"At first, I was afraid I would get hurt again, but now I know Sov listens, watches out for me and takes good care of me." J.M., Seattle, WA

Chapter Three

Too Close To The Forest

Being "too close to the forest to see the trees" applies to the emotions related to weight loss, because without awareness of self, people tend to experience emotions without having perspective on them [*as they are having them*]. A typical scenario most of us can relate to is saying someone has a temper...once something triggers them they can't get perspective and cool down until much later, if at all. Part of taking responsibility is noticing your triggers before they trigger you, then interrupt the reaction all together, giving yourself more choices about your behaviors. The key being to "notice".

A similar pattern repeats itself with regard to weight loss in that the emotions get triggered, usually outside of awareness, until someone develops self-awareness (introspection) and goes about intervening on their own patterns by learning to notice what sets them off/triggers them and then through repetitively noticing themselves and what came right before they got triggered.

Each time you learn to notice what "set off"/triggered a series of unconscious responses, which lead to unwanted behaviors (like binging on junk food), you've effectively bridged the gap between having goals, but then unconsciously interrupt, doing self-sabotage behavior and then wondering, *"How that could happen?"*

By consciously repeating the process you become or "make conscious" the patterns that, up until then, had been happening outside your awareness (unconsciously)/habitually.

So, you see how personal accountability is important since no trainer or health care provider for that matter can be with you 24 hours a day and even if they could you would still have to do it yourself...*you have to be present with yourself.*

Now, you can see that for much of the population, getting overweight and being overweight is a gradual, but [predictable] process of being unaware of your own emotional triggers, which engage you to push emotions down, then consume in such a way to use your energy to keep the emotions suppressed, *then disassociate from them and forget how you got like that* (habit).

One of the most effective ways to become aware of your own patterns is when you notice yourself behaving/doing something that is not in alignment with your goals, but you can't seem to stop, take a deep breath, notice your breath and ask yourself, *"What came before this?"* and then wait/be patient to receive an answer. You don't have to stop the thing, at first, *just notice it.* Be aware of it.

You have to be open to whatever answer you get whether it's a picture, words or feelings. What is likely to happen is your mind/body will communicate with you the best it can, but it might surprise you how it goes about it. You might see yourself, in your mind's eye, having whatever experience just triggered a conditioned emotional response that was similar to the first time it happened.

For example, I had a client who talked about when she was a child and whether she got in a disagreement with her parents or something happened that made her feel down or sad, she would run to her room with a package of cookies or chips and eat the whole package. The S.A.D.C.R.A.P. being an effective means to feel better (disassociate from the pain), in the short-run, but gain immense fat in the long run. Once it worked to relieve her emotional pain the first time, it became a crutch/anchor for her. In examining herself the way I describe above *("What came before this?")* she realized she had continued this on for 40 years and even shopped for S.A.D.C.R.A.P. to have on hand in case she experienced any pain on any given day, as though it were medication.

A powerful tip here is that once you get the answer of what came before, it might be enough self-awareness to provide adequate insight to curb your emotional reaction...the simple act of a little more self-awareness can be very healing. At various times in my own life where I was changing my knee-jerk, emotional reactions, after I got the first answer I would say, *"Ok, got it, what came before that!?"*

Repeating this, in place of impulsive emotional reactions, or trying to suppress the behaviors or judge it, can be repeated until you trace your reactions back to one of the original sources of the emotional driver...the point where for lack of better coping mechanisms, a choice to proceed in a way that relieved the discomfort in the moment, but left to its own, hinders health and wellness in the long-run...*also known as a form of self-sabotage.*

Changing habits can be as easy as simply forcing yourself to do a healthier version of a habit, e.g. exercising versus being inactive.

Generally speaking, new habits or replacement habits take about three weeks of consistent application for it to take on a life of its own as a healthier lifestyle (to the point where you feel "off" if you don't complete the task). And for people who don't have the conflicting emotional pains, they are the ones who take to an exercise program and nutrition program and run with it without interruption. Even with athletes or anyone successful at their exercise program, there's always days when you have to talk yourself into doing your workout...*that's self-discipline.*

In regard to new habits for a healthier lifestyle, it's not uncommon for people to be in a routine and everything is going fine, but when they change the context (location or circumstances) where they are doing their workouts and nutritional habits they fall off the wagon and revert to reactive, unhealthy habits. So, you have to make a plan for unexpected changes in routine...*nip it* ahead of time. Changes occur to everyone, so the antidote is to simply plan on them happening.

Falling-off-the-wagon or regressing/reverting simply points to [deeper aspects] of unresolved emotions. People tend to be able to clean up various aspects of their pain in one environment and when they go into another environment they are particularly vulnerable to having other triggers they weren't conscious of getting triggered. Its kinda' like life says, *"You've done good so far, let's up the ante."* It happens to everyone, so you have to build it into your plan. If you don't acknowledge the potential that I told you it will happen, then it will come as some surprise and you wan't be prepared. Now you know.

As we grow, develop and improve in a certain context, life will offer you the opportunities to expand on your emotional development. Each time this cycle happens, you let go of a little more pain, replace it with a little more competency and develop yourself-image as a fit person a little more. It's at this point that you'll begin having others ask you to help them and you pay it forward.

Chapter conclusion:

The greatest skill you can cultivate is becoming aware of your emotions and what occurred before you experienced those emotions. By practicing this, you effectively short-circuit the emotional states which were previously sabotaging your efforts.

Plan on life-interruptions, in your routine and have plans in place to deal with changes, so you're not tempted to say you couldn't find any healthy food, didn't remember to take your supplements, forgot your functional-food drinks or didn't know what to do with your workouts.

Left to their own, without intervention, imbalanced emotions can become influencers of the mental capacity and the mental capacity can affect overall quality of health outcomes. Meaning, if you don't manage your emotions, when you have the chance, the emotions affect physological processes and those affect physical health/weight/body composition through information-transduction (the brain taking ideas and converting them into brain chemicals/neuro-transmitters), which in-turn control behaviors: The well-nourished brain craves healthy, whole-foods and has the hands grab heathier choices. The under-nourished brain craves SADCRAP, makes choices based on immediate, emotional-satisfaction and has the hands grab SADCRAP, thereby sabotaging consistency in weight loss efforts.

No single, greater factor influences and helps assure weight loss success than consistent, correct application of the B.N.B.B.s, *without substitution.*

"I have taken what I learned from you here about training enough, but not too much…you know leaving some energy for recovery and have been applying it to the rest of my life including my work at [the major software company]…I believe it's my new super-power."
J.R., Seattle, WA

Chapter Four

The Natural Laws of Emotional Responsibility

"A negative situation can empower you if you're willing to do what it takes to create balance."

Cesar Millan, *The Dog Whisperer*

There are what I refer to, for lack of better terms, as the natural-laws of emotional responsibility. These are patterns I have noticed as to what happens and what the implications are for people who manage their own emotions and take responsibility for them, as well as what happens when people either ignore their responsibility or attempt to get others to take responsibility for their emotions...*lacking coping skills for the pain they perceive they are experiencing* (having feelings).

One example of this would be the spouse who constantly complains about their spouse not doing enough, earning enough, being enough or generally, just being a complete disappointment to them (trainers, like bartenders, *hear it all*...especially since a lot of people get personal training to get away from their spouse). People who misunderstand the natural laws of emotional responsibility don't understand that what you focus on grows...so if your focus is on how inadequate your spouse is you're actually inviting and manifesting (directly or indirectly) more of what you insist you don't want. The more you complain about your spouse (to them and to family and friends, about them), the less likely you are to feel satisfied by your spouse and the less likely your spouse will feel inclined to go out of their way to help you feel satisfied.

The words "edify" (to instruct, especially so as to encourage intellectual, moral and/or spiritual improvement) and "honor" (honesty, fairness & respect) for your spouse, come to mind.

More often than not, people who constantly complain about their spouse are essentially screaming for help to escape the hell they have co-created for themselves, where they have co-created a prison of combined low self-esteem & lack of confidence (lack of personal accomplishment), lack of independence (overtly dependent on their spouse for emotional support, whom they don't respect) and/or insecurity (inadequate/under developed self-image). When people are unhappy with themselves, instead of taking a deep breath, asking a question, getting quiet and being patient for the answer, they look outside themselves (instead of inside) and blame those they are closest and most comfortable with, for the feelings they are having in that moment...in essence, screaming, *"Fix me! Fix what I'm feeling!"* When people have strong feelings and they don't attend to them themselves they focus on what they insist is wrong with other people, instead of figuring themselves out...which make two people unhappy.

People who insist on this type of inappropriate expression, will often attempt to seek out and surround themselves with people who also love to complain about others rather than improving themselves (co-miserating). Sometimes, it's a simple lack of understanding that complaining and problem solving/brain-storming are two different behaviors (based on intention). It's not as imbalanced to get together with people who mutually care for each other and tell you situation and come from a place of asking, *"What do you guys do in this situation?"* or *"What does this mean?"* or *"What is my role in the situation"*, but if you find yourself attempting to take people to lunch just to have a bitch-session about all that is wrong with your spouse...*well, let's just say co-miserating will get you more of what you insist you don't want* and you might be so caught up in attempting to defame your spouse that you're not really aware of how you are appearing and sounding to those around you.

Essentially, life offers two choices...you can either play the victim/wounded/martyr/disempowered/lemons role or you can play the victor/rise-to-the-occasion/empower yourself/confessor/lemonade role, but when you try to play both roles, you exhaust and deplete yourself, limiting your choices and losing all your friends...if you do have people continue to meet with you to hear your complaining, it's out of pity, not out of commonality or camaraderie.

People who are stuck in the misery mindset misunderstand that it's up to them to change/improve their situation...to keep complaining about your spouse says more about you than it does them, since you're effectively claiming you don't have any control over your situation nor any respect for you or your spouse. Again, problem solving is not the same as venting or explaining the situation to brain-storm solutions. Over the decades I've had a few clients stuck in this downward cycle, a common dynamic is them seeking out counselors who will agree with them but not help them figure out or disclose where they are contributing to the problem. If they do find a counselor who is straight up with them, they don't go back, complaining they don't like the counselor's "style". But, that's the point of complaining about the spouse (distracting themselves from their *dis*-satisfaction with themselves), insisting on being "right" all the time in every situation (you can be right or loved: *you choose*) and surrounding themselves with people who agree with them, even when they aren't right or rational.

In order for a person to escape this cycle, they'll have to increase focus on introspection (examination of one's own conscious thoughts and feelings: in psychology the process of introspection relies exclusively on observation of one's mental and emotional states; closely related to human self-reflection).

People who insist that their viewpoint is the only valid one and any discussion with others is to simply convince others of your viewpoint are essentially eliminating room in their life for people, other than themselves. If you have to "be right" to feel right, your self-esteem is in the gutter, completely under developed. The stronger a person's self-esteem, the more difference and diversity you can tolerate. If you're going to counseling just to have a professional listen to you cry and complain then tell you you're ok and right, it's the rest of the world that is wrong, you just got suckered out of your money and the point of counseling or therapy may be lost on you.

A major point of therapy is to improve yourself through introspection. And yes, there's a million different models, I'm talking about effective, consistent, sustainable weight loss. If you simply want to vent, then tell the therapist you don't want to change, you just want to vent...at least then you're being honest with yourself. The idea is to find the counselor/therapist who will call you out on your poop, but whom you feel comfortable with enough to take it in and stick with it even if it's not as comfortable as a bitch session with acquaintances...that's how you get help from counseling...not by insisting to be told you're right. Hear the distinction?

A common phrase people who insist on being right all the time is, *"Yay, I'm just saying..."* and they repeat the thing back thinking that if they repeat their point enough times, you'll agree with them. People who repeat the same thing over and over are wanting to be heard because they perceive they aren't being heard, even when people have already heard it over and over...often for decades…which means they aren't listening to themselves, but subsequently projecting the "non-hearing" to those around themselves.

One of the diagnostic tools used in the mental health realms is whether or not a person's story can be intervened on. In other words, if a person cannot entertain other possibilities and an outsider can't affect their story or perception at all, it's one of many indicators of various types of mental illness, but that doesn't apply to most people.

Most people, as they improve themselves and take their focus off what's wrong with others, find it less important to be right all the time. A Catch-22 here, is if a person is superstitious or so deeply lacks understanding and deeply believes that it makes them a bad person if they aren't right all the time. In this case, it's very difficult to intervene (help the person improve), since the person is wrapped up in circular-logic, in that they are inhibiting their own progress and personal development, but they have built psychological perimeters to prevent anyone from interacting with the dynamic they complain about, yet resist change or improvement of (double-bind).

So, in essence, the person is complaining about their spouse, but have set it up so if anyone tells them it isn't about their spouse, the eliminate them from their circle of influence in favor of people who will seem to sympathize with them. Sometimes, the whole process is a guise to gain energy from others. When balance is in place, people gain good energy from exercise, nutrition and spiritual practices as well as being out in nature (the forest and ocean). But, people who haven't been consistent with these, engage in melodrama to manipulate other's energy through sympathy and having others feel sorry for them. These people often jump from one church to another, once again, discounting others once the group, as a whole, catches on to their pattern (lack of introspection and blaming others for their unhappiness).

If it was really about the problem they say it is, they would have changed the dynamic long ago, unless they are too deficient to recognize the situation they have co-created.

More often than not, when a couple is having a power-struggle or simply not getting along, it's an indicator (albeit discreet) that it's time for personal growth, either for one person or both...but you can't make a person seek self-improvement...it's an inside job. When a couple isn't "meshing" (especially if one person is impatient with their spouse), it's a good indicator that the spouse who is the most "troubled" [by the other] needs to improve themselves, most often by improving their energy level through exercise, nutrition and spiritual practices (when a person has low energy and doesn't realize their *dis*-sastisfaction is rooted with themselves). I'm not talking about being troubled by an abusive person, but rather one person being so bothered by anothers' personal choices or how they arrange their daily routine.

What we "civilized" people tend to overlook or forget once we're in a committed relationship is that in nature, beings (regardless of classification) with more energy or personal power tend to attract others...others with higher energy. Self-confidence, self-assurance, self-satisfaction and fulfillment tend to attract others. Negative, complainers tend to push people away. The negative person, who believes they are positive is a whole different deal.

In relationships, power struggles aren't from two powerful-in-their-own-right people fighting for position, but rather from trying to get the other person to do something they don't want to or not motivated to do. BUT, if you simply focus on improving your own natural energy level (the kind you get from exercise, nutrition and some sort of spiritual practice [not necessarily religion]), the "power" struggle seems to mellow out or dissolve. I've seen this often where if one or both people start focusing on improving themselves they each start remembering and refocusing on what they liked about each other to begin with. In other words, a false power struggle is when each person is simply focusing too much on what they find fault with in their partner. When they take away finding fault and refocus on improving themselves, they begin feeling physically, mentally and emotionally better and don't seem to have a need to criticize others any more...then their self-worth compass is pointed closer to true North, since they are attracted to feeling better from working out and eating better rather than pulling energy away from other people. I had a boss one time that called these kinds of people energy-vampires or time-gremlins, since they want to take up your time, the conversation doesn't really end up anywhere productive and you feel tired and exhausted after being around them.

An example of this is when someone *dis*-associates from their own emotions to the extent that when they have a feeling inside, whether it is random or triggered by others, instead of taking a deep breath, bringing their attention down inside where the feeling seems to be located and asking, *"What that's about?"* they instead look around for the nearest person and erroneously conclude the feeling is about the other person....constantly bouncing from one drama and disappointment to another and not understanding why they are having such a hard time.

How a person develops this immature and incomplete pattern often comes from some peer(s) modeling the same behaviors to them...not taking responsibility for their emotions and then blaming those around them for the emotions they don't know how to handle. Remember how we learn ways of being, long before we know we're even learning? People generally exhibit how they were treated by treating others the same ways (lack of introspection and unresolved pain), but not always.

As long as a person tries to escape feelings that aren't comfortable instead of being curious and inquiring with themselves about them, they'll continue to blame others for how they feel, but the flip side is that they will likely believe that being truly happy is also outside their control...happiness only comes from the spouse or others doing what pleases you...you can't have it both ways...Are you powerful and in control of your life? Or are you a powerless weakling destined for unhappiness?

I believe, as I said earlier that the point of emotions is to enhance whatever experiences we have in life...to bring greater intensity to pleasurable experiences as well as give us feedback (gut-feelings) when something is amiss. But when we push negative experiences down/suppress, in order to avoid reliving the previous pain we might subsequently experience anxiety and depression. Suppression of feelings rather than expression and release uses energy that could be used to simply do exercise and nutrition. The subsequent consequences or flip side is we're so busy keeping old stuff at bay that we can't be present enough to thoroughly enjoy current times...life seems to lack a little luster and often we then conclude that nothing will give us any more pleasure than what we are currently having suppressing old content down. How happy is that?

These kinds of decisions, at least at first, are being made at the unconscious level. Once we earn to communicate with ourselves to figure them out instead of letting the emotions run us the way they did earlier we begin to have clearer and more genuine responses and life becomes more enjoyable and takes on new meaning.

Chapter conclusion:

Life seems to give people who complain more things and greater intensity of the things they complain about. Life seems to give people who practice gratitude more of that they say they are grateful for, *even if they didn't have any of it to begin with.* What you focus on grows. If you can't control what you focus on, you could benefit from practicing focus. There's plenty of positive, successful, satisfied, fulfilled people to model until you get the hang of it and teach others. If you allow yourself to be distracted, it's likely you'll continue to struggle to reach your goals let alone maintain them.

The hunger center of the brain is regulated, based on the quantity of nutrition you have in your body/brain, compared to what you personally need. The higher your nutrition level, the more regulated hunger and cravings are. Food and nutrition are, for this sake, considered two very different things. When you have enough nutrition, there are no cravings for unhealthy S.A.D.C.R.A.P.

"If anyone wants to know what you are like as a trainer, have them call and speak to me personally...I would not have purchased more training now I will." J.B., Seattle, WA

Chapter Five

Self-awareness Is Paramount

Up until this point, in the book, I've used the term [weight loss], but what we're really talking about is [fat-loss]. The reason being is that weight loss is not a focus of *health first*, its primary focus is on what the scale says...*a number that has nothing to do with your overall health*. Hopefully you know this already and it's not new information. There are some cases where people are clinically obese (an example of body-fat of 30% or more), and getting the weight down is an urgent, high-priority on the path to health. But, if these terms aren't clarified from the get-go, misunderstandings will likely occur and most people will still have health problems (high blood sugar, high cholesterol, etc.) even though the scale says the weight decreased. Your initial body-fat percentage goal (body composition) should be 20% or less (more on this later).

If someone has resistance to or behaves offended by the term fat-loss, it indicates an emotional sticking-point, related to denial of their situation. If a person can't name that they are on a fat-loss journey, they're essentially in denial about where they are and what actions have to be taken. Until one can say they are working to decrease their fat they haven't come to terms with the seriousness of their situation (more than 20% body-fat). If this is the case, it hints as to where attention needs to be paid in terms of updating their language and awareness to match their current goals. A great indicator of whether someone has really made the decision to reach their goals is whether they can speak the language that matches that of a person who intends to follow through and succeed, versus coming up against their previous limitations and backing off again.

One of author George Orwell's quotes, *"Control the language and you control the people,"* applies here, it's just that when you control your language you begin to take control of your own life...a lot of personal trainers can estimate how committed and likely a person is to reach their short and long-term goals based on the language clients use…even during the initial consulation/interview. The reason for this is that the words, phrases and metaphors a person express can indicate a person's beliefs, values and commitment level, even outside their own awareness. Self-awareness includes listening to yourself because it indicates things about your own mind set that you might not be conscious of yourself! (introspection).

If a person doesn't learn enough about themselves to dial-in and refine their efforts to decrease body-fat exclusively and increase lean mass and all the markers of health (cholesterol, blood pressure, iron, triglycerides, HDL, LDL, blood sugar, etc.), they will not necessarily improve even though their "weight" has decreased...*you can't fool nature!* The problem being that when people are focusing on losing "weight" they don't know if they lost any fat versus a loss of lean tissue, bone density and organ mass. The people who are watching the scale exclusively and watching their clothing size are some of the most likely to *not* sustain or maintain their body composition improvements...their focus and self-awareness are not in the right places.

Sustainable fat-loss is the result of participating in the process (resistance-training, fat-burning cardio and the three points of nutrition), and simply continuing the process, *refining as you go.* If you see it as a thing you'll do one time or for a time, you won't maintain your success nor be satisfied with the results. *It's a lifestyle!* People who focus on the scale, or how many "inches" they lost or how many clothing sizes they have decreased generally gain all the weight back and more, since they haven't taken the responsibility to learn about optimizing their health and becoming healthier as time goes on...*self-awareness.*

By focusing on the scale, clothing size or inches lost the more likely you'll lose lean mass and the more body-fat they'll gain back once you've have pushed their body to the point where it can't afford to lose any more lean mass (lean mass being muscle, bone, tendon, organs...*everything except fat*) and the nutritional resources have been used up from activity. A reason for this is that from an emotional perspective, people who focus on the scale number, inches lost or clothing size are looking at weight loss as a quick fix to an unhealthy lifestyle, rather than a process or lifestyle. The most satisfied people are the ones who focus on living a fitness-lifestyle and understand that it's a process rather than a quick fix way to reverse chronic poor choices in food and activity. The people who think they can achieve a quick fix, as if there aren't consequences for poor nutritional habits and exercise don't maintain any weight loss, since they think they can just diet and reverse the consequences willy-nilly. People who don't focus on the process through a fitness-lifestyle (which is very fun and satisfying) usually skip updating their resting heart rate, body composition and caloric requirements, the first of each month...*hint, hint*. When you drive your car or truck you have to fuel up ahead of time for obvious reasons and the body is the same way.

So, from this point forward I'll be referring to [fat-loss] instead of weight loss. Fat-loss indicates the body has begun to tap into body-fat as an energy source, ultimately getting to a point where you're burning fat for energy even when you're sleeping...*an average fat-loss every 24 hours and 30 days...*this is how you can wake up and have lost five or six pounds over night...not every night, but as the body builds up adequate nutritional density surplus, the body releases the equivalent body-fat. *But, the nutrition density has to be on board, first!*

To do this, you have to learn about what makes your body run efficiently and what gets in the way of your body running efficiently. Remember, healthy fat-loss comes down to a combination of resistance-training, strategic fat-burning, cardiovascular-training and optimized nutrition: 1) Whole-foods, 2) Functional-foods and 3) Certain dietary supplements at certain times to fill in the gaps (B.N.B.B.s). Skip a part, from the beginning, and you simply won't get the quality results you could have. People who procrastinate or skip steps or parts of a program often wonder why they are doing all the work but not getting results (a side effect of inadequate nutrition), the often get injured or start having health problems and burn out within three to five months of beginning their program.

At a certain point, in order to have continued and sustainable success you have to become self-aware. The more self-aware you become the easier, more efficient and more effective your progress will be...you take each lesson you learn and apply it to future which results in cumulative benefits (meaning you may go three days without burning any fat, but then wake up in the morning five pounds lighter). The people you see who are lean, healthy, happy and fulfilled have gotten that way partly by being aware of themselves and what makes their body burn fat efficiently and consistently

Some people start out with emotional imbalances that interfere with their progress and some people are emotionally clear to begin with, but either way allowing the emotions to run the show prevents progress and interferes with momentum. Part of the reason people who seem so happy and so evangelistic about fitness is because it feels so good to be fit and healthy and be in control of your mind, body and emotions...they *want others to experience the same things!* People who are fit and healthy tend to have a sense of control over their lives as opposed to gaining a sense of control through consuming S.A.D.C.R.A.P., refusing to exercise properly and consistently, as well as consciously withholding the B.N.B.B.s./failing to put the B.N.B.B.s in your body.

A common problem seen in gyms and by trainers is when people over-identify with their negative emotions, meaning they think they *are* their emotions (or don't know there's other ways of being). This characteristic is often noticed a person who identifies with their negative emotions are around someone who is light-hearted and very positive; it reflects back to them as though they can't stand to improve themselves. When someone [over identifies] with their emotions they feel more "right" when they are experiencing emotions, *even if the emotions themselves are depressing and a major downer* (familiarity)...they are attached to the emotions that are supposed to be experienced and let go! This is not unlike the pattern of the habitual complainer who leads or redirects every conversation to what isn't right...they've done it so much it feels normal. People who have the most difficult time simply doing exercise and nutrition are effectively putting their focus on maintaining their link/connection to emotions which are getting in their way, since the emotions feel so familiar, even though they are unproductive and interfering with their mental clarity and physical energy and motivation.

The person who [over identifies with their feelings] and doesn't know there's the option not to, may perceive that people are saying something is wrong with them, as opposed to seeing people are helping them refine their process of fat-loss. Remember, emotions are supposed to enhance your life experiences...*they aren't supposed to be the experience itself...they aren't supposed to be the container of your identity.* When a person finally makes the conscious distinction that they can *experience* emotions, but they aren't supposed/don't have to *be* their emotions, they generally describe a feeling of a *weight being lifted* and as though they *can do anything now* (not being held down by feelings)...as though they thought they had a responsibility to carry those emotions (the boat anchor affect of junk food), as described earlier.

The people who have an advantage in this are the ones who have mentors, trainers, friends or even family members who demonstrated being self-aware versus being disassociated or "checked-out". Experiencing emotions versus *being* emotions can happen by conscious decision (if there is enough self-awareness) or by watching and modeling people who seem light on their feet and light-hearted, *looking forward to a bright future*. Athletes and anyone involved in athletic activities of any kind also have the advantage since they learned alone the way to set the feelings about the situation aside, in order to get the bigger goal in the moment. You have to effectively take charge of your mind, versus letting the mind happen and then behaving as if you didn't have any say in it.

If you spend any time around successful athletes, you'll notice that any time they happen upon a negative person, they simply move away...they don't even discuss it, since negative people tend to want to justify their negativity by engaging in negative conversation (major energy waster and distraction). Some people are so rooted in negativity, that to even have a conversation with them is a negative expereince. You'll notice that successful athletes rarely talk about being sick or what isn't working, since they already know that what they focus on grows. Athletes will use injury or illness as an indicator of where they need to improve, focus on fundamentals, take better care of themselves or refine their habits, but they don't attempt to gain attention, sympathy or create bonds with others based on injury or illness...it's all distraction from being healthy.

Resisting the natural laws of nature:

Another challenging phenomena seen is with the people who resist the natural laws of cause-and-effect...*do the thing, get the effect*. People who didn't realize the quality of experiences they have been having all along in life (for better or worse) is related to their emotional state. These people have a difficult time letting go of negative, unproductive emotions since there tend to be a part of them that wants to have their cake and eat it too!..meaning, they want to indulge in entertaining the familiar guests of negativity, self-loathing and depressive feelings, but get the reward of people who generate positive, generative, productive emotions...*hint, hint. You can generate positive emotions without having an external reason to do so!* The side effects include a brighter outlook, a feeling as though a wait has been lifted and a feeling that you can accomplish anything! The most simple way to do this is to remember times when you experienced positive emotions before. At any moment, you can begin generating the emotions which fuel your success...weighting for positive emotions to happen is wackbards thinking!

One of those challenging emotional attitudes that trainers and all medical personnel have is that of the person who doesn't want the laws of nature to apply to them...*they resist what is*...they insist they are *the* one exception to the rule. There are a couple really important reasons for this dynamic that I want you to get and take in to make your own journey easier and more efficient. The first being the non-negotiable law of nutrition and its effects on the brain, the mind and the emotions in relation to Fat-loss.

There is no single greater factor that helps a person get their mind and emotions in the right place to make progress and sustain progress than the *amount, quantity, quality and timing* of nutrition density a person consumes on a daily basis or misses out on (more on this later). In other words, a person may insist they want help with their attitude, emotions and physical well-being, but then simply refuse to do the three nutrition parts (they say they want help, but refuse to do the thing). Beginners often don't realize that the really fit, well-nourished, well-adjusted training clients get that way by putting the nutrition in their body, even though they don't feel like it or it doesn't make sense...*hint, hint...you won't feel like it or understand it until you do it consistently enough to get measurable results* (one to three months to begin with a one year commitment). If you aren't willing to do it for a full year, then don't start...you haven't decided, committed nor are you ready to follow through (more on this in the six stages to behavioral change).

Steps in the right direction:

Self-awareness is a vast topic. If you imagine the yogis of India who can do all sorts of superhuman feats, you get the idea to the extent one can take self-awareness. In the context of fat-loss, you don't have to take it *that* far. I'm primarily talking about underlying motivations...*why you do what you do, in the context of burning fat,* getting lean, taking control of your health and then going on to sustaining your progress. It really comes down to asking yourself, *"What came before this?"*

People who tend to [lack control] over their nutrition and exercise tend to [react] emotionally, basically bouncing from one reaction to another to avoid uncomfortable feelings (instead of moving toward what they do want to experience)...a form of escapism which is usually accompanied by behaviors that get them the opposite of what their goals are. Without self-awareness, the knee-jerk reactions go unchecked and the net result is accumulation of gained body-fat, albeit slow but consistently. They generally aren't aware of what made them want to change their emotional state, suppress the feelings or avoid life's stresses in general. One of the greatest keys to self-awareness is to simply watch, listen and/or feel what the thing was...without reacting to it...just notice it. Positive emotional states are more a matter of focusing on positive emotions (often from positive experiences), then practicing enough that it become an unconscious habit. Easy!

The concept of getting "present" is the underlying quality for any goal or self-improvement program because we learn ways of dealing with stress, life and disappointments generally before we know we're learning. Ultimately, you could trace it back to choices, but as children we're rarely conscious enough to project the long-term implications of our choices. When I was a kid I suffered with low blood sugar and anemia a lot. The side effect was that I would get ravenous and very shaky and run to the cookie can and scarf as much as I could to try to get my blood sugar back up. Ultimately, the sugar rushes from being malnourished and then consuming S.A.D.C.R.A.P. really took a toll on my digestive, immune and circulatory systems. Around the seventh or eighth grade I began associating getting sick all the time with the amount of sugar I was consuming and related the constant sore throat to all the refined sugars I was eating. Until that moment I was clueless to the cause and affect of what I was putting in my body. *What came before this!?*

So, the point is that there's no secret magic to self-awareness, it simply comes down to acknowledging there might be other options of ways to be in the world and once you become curious about what came before doing a behavior that you really would rather have control over, ask yourself, *"What came before this?"* Then be patient and wait for the answer to come in whatever way it comes (auditory, visual or feeling). When you do get the answer, say, *"Thank you"* to make conscious something that has been an unconscious process and to acknowledge to yourself that you had some insight.

If you don't notice an answer at first, it doesn't mean anything other than you're working on getting tuned-in to your own self-awareness. People who have been avoiding painful or stressful content/details generally have been operating out of an ego/survival/self-preservation/defensive state of mind and what is needed is to set the ego aside, get quiet and be present...*make room for the answers that will release you from your past.* Generally, when given a choice, and knowing there is something else available (the payoff of reaching your goals), people let go of what hasn't been working for what will definitely take you to your goals.

Chapter conclusion:

Change your ideas and the way you speak about weight loss to fat-loss. The body is the tangible container of the intangible things we refer to as emotions (much like what the mind is to the brain). Your primary goal is to experience emotions to enhance your life experiences, then let them go! By letting emotions go, instead of holding them in, staying on track with your exercise and nutrition is easy...you'll automatically have more energy and clarity. If you're struggling to stay on track with you exercise and nutrition: 1) Whole-foods 2) Functional-foods and 3) Certain dietary supplements at certain times (B.N.B.B.s), the emotions are getting in the way (non-productive emotional state).

"You are different than my other trainer ...you are professional."
J.G., Seattle, WA

Chapter Six

There Are No Secrets
To Healthy Fat-loss Anymore

Probably the most common question trainers get from people who are desperate to burn fat is, *"What's the secret to fat-loss?"*

There's good news and bad news to this. The bad news is that there isn't a "secret". The good news is that the reason there's no secret to fat-loss is because its already been figured out. The people who are just starting their journey rely heavy on learning the "science" of fat-loss. As you master the fundamentals (exercise and nutrition), specifically resistance-training combined with some strategic, fat-burning cardiovascular/aerobic training, combined with a three-part, complete nutrition program (as described), *patterns* emerge.

By continuing to rely on the fundamentals as the basis of your program and then expanding on it, by introducing variations here and there (hopefully with guidance), the art of burning fat emerges and then fine-tuning comes into play as you maintain/sustain the progress you've made...the "art" being paying attention to notice nuances with your own body (like, *"I feel better if I eat every three hours versus every five hours"*). How will your life be different when you are lean and healthy?

For example, the "constant" is having enough nutrition [and] food on board prior to your workouts, but whether you eat up until your workout or stop eating a half an hour before your workout (based on your digestion and blood sugar levels) is the "art" part. You can't skimp on calories, but the timing, to some extent will be unique to you as long as you get enough calories. It's like saying everyone uses water to get clean, but the temperature you prefer is up to you and whether or not you burn your skin or cool down.

For the seasoned trainer, there are no mysteries nor unknowns in relation to fat-loss. There's nothing a new client can say that will either baffle, confuse or distract a trainer since the fundamentals are already proven (it's not uncommon for people who insist they need to lose weight to spend hours each night on the web researching the "secrets to fat-loss" but insisting they don't have time for exercise and even if they did, they might reply *"...exercise doesn't help me"*). When they are presented with a proven plan, they insite they haven't heard of it.

I guess if there was a secret, it would be that your life story is unique to you, but the things you'll do to burn fat and get lean are fundamentally the same for everyone...you're just not so unique that a whole new program has to be designed for you to burn fat. If you have convinced yourself of this, notice that it's a distraction and a way to procrastinate, discount and dismiss what definitely works.

One of the consistent emotional challenges that comes up in this scenario is when people insist that their situation is so "different". In order to keep the content of their past suppressed and outside [their] awareness they insist that their situation is different and no one can understand them. This is such a biased viewpoint because they are in so much denial, using so much energy to contain their emotions in the container called body-fat that they have convinced [themselves] that no one else knows the content of their past...what they don't get is that no one needs to nor has to understand that stuff in order for them to do the resistance training, the cardiovascular training and sticking to the nutrition plan...*the science of fat-loss.*

The greatest challenge I've consistently seen with almost every single fat-loss client in over thirty years...even people I was training before I was certified, is to simply keep moving (doing the exercise you're scheduled to) regardless of what you are emotionally feeling. Emotions are relevant when they are empowering you to do the behaviors of exercise and nutrition. But, more often than not, negative emotions intend to keep us from experiencing more pain, but since they are rooted in the past (out of context and not related to present time), they gradually take over more and more of our being, essentially shutting us down and limiting our experience to the point of feeling paralyzed. The result being we have difficulty knowing exactly what to pay atnetion to and what to filter out (false skepticism).

The single greatest road block to fat-loss is convincing yourself that because you're having feelings, you can't/won't continue working out. The best tip I have is to simply keep moving, until the emotional-content (feelings) move out of your body the way they are naturally supposed to, instead of freezing up and behaving as if having feelings is an indicator to stop moving and start consuming S.A.D.C.R.A.P.

Whether someone knows your story, understands your life or not, it still comes down to you doing the behavior of the science of fat-loss. The science of fat-loss is the constant that doesn't change no matter what your story is, no matter what you believe, no matter what someone knows or doesn't know about you. Like Nike says, *Just Do It!* Yes, you should get a check-up with your physician and medical team prior to beginning an exercise and nutrition program to make sure there aren't contraindications that have to be addressed [before you begin].

Chapter conclusion:

There's no "secret" to fat-loss, as long as your exrcise program and nutritional program is specifically designed for your current health status, body composition level, your current fitness level and what your primary and secondary goals are. Nutrition is a higher priority than exercise and nutrition density is a higher priority than caloric-reduction. Eating excess calories is a symptom of too little nutrition density (B.N.B.B.s in the brain). Cravings S.A.D.C.R.A.P. over healthier food is also a symptom of inadequate B.N.B.B.s. You have to prioritize the [three parts] of nutrition and proper activity, in your life and [follow through]. If I was pushed to say theire's a secret, it would be that we aren't aware of what we aren't aware of… and you won't be fully aware until you have adequate nutrition in your brain, fueling/activating the front of the brain, and down-playing the limbic/emotional aspect of the brain, which is rooted in how well you apply the B.N.B.B.s./how well-nourished your brain is. The under-nourished person will not have enough nutrition density to be aware enough to stick to any program about anything. The undernousished-brain cannot take in the very information (about nutrition) that would effectively save its own life.

Generally speaking, the more resisatnt a person is to the B.N.B.B.s, the more they need them.

"You don't just do personal training…you bring all your skills to the sessions and people's lives change quickly." L.I., Seattle, WA

Chapter Seven

The *Catch-22* of Fat-Loss

I promised I would talk about how nutrition plays into the mind/body/emotional link.

Over the past thirty-plus years I've helped people at all different levels. Some people wanted help to lose the last few pounds, some were athletes wanting to improve their strength-to-weight ratio, some were just beginning the journey at 50% of their body composition being fat and their doctor telling them they'll die prematurely if they don't get in shape. Sometimes people have health considerations that have to be taken into account in designing their program. The common denominator with every one of them was deficiency in their strategy and application of nutrition. There's many reasons for this, mostly related to a misunderstanding of what nutrition means and partly because there is so much conflicting information out there (which I cover in detail).

The quick-and-dirty of what definitely works (the science of solid, effective nutrition), is a combination of 1) Whole-foods, 2) Functional-foods and 3) Certain dietary supplements at certain times (to fill in the nutritional gaps everyone experiences as a part of living). If you're serious about burning fat, don't leave it to chance. Leave no stone unturned. Nutritional gaps definitely prevent the liberation of body-fat for energy (also known as a plateau, *"I can't lose weight".*).

The Catch-22 of fat-loss is that cardiovascular exercise (cycling, rowing, running, walking, swimming), will burn fat, but without adequate nutrition: 1) Whole-foods, 2) Functional-foods and 3) Certain dietary supplements at certain times, you'll unfortunately be unable to retain your lean mass...the only way to know if you're getting enough nutrition to retain your lean mass is through monitoring your body composition the first of each month (30 day average). But without certain supplements at the correct times, by the time you realize you're deficient, you've already hit a plateau in progress, regardless how much you increase your exercise intensity, frequency or duration. Without supplementation, the more you exercise the more lean mass you'll lose.

Without proper supplementation, you're unwittingly wasting time, energy and money…spinning your wheels. A lot of people who seem malnourished seem to enjoy arguing about nutrition. An argumentative attitude is common with undernourishment, especially extra B vitamins. But the science doesn't lie. You can debate whether food has enough nutrition all you want. The scientific way to know is whether or not you're retaining and gaining lean mass, bone density and experiencing improvements in your blood chemistry numbers. A person who isn't nourished, will struggle to get their blood chemistry numbers in the healthy zone, regardless how healthy they insist they eat or how much nutrition they argue is in whatever food they choose. Body composition is a great indicator when people insist they are getting enough nutrition from food alone. Time and time again (and you may have seen this phenomena in your own life) people consult a person they identify as an expert, but they already have their mind made up about what they are willing/unwilling to do, before they ever get to their expert appointment.

What I generally do with these kinds of personalities is show them the criteria for how to know if their nutrition program is actually providing measurable improvement (body composition and blood chemistry lab panel) and ask them if what they are doing is providing those scientific improvements. The reason being, that if your body composition (ratio of lean mass to body-fat), isn't improving you're essentially depriving your body (of nutritional density) and any results will be short-lived. Secondly, the basis of any real, health-first, health building fat-loss program has to be health first...*the blood chemistry panel is the definitive guide for underlying health or lack thereof.* A nutrition program that doesn't improve the blood chemistry and body composition is not a nutrition program, it's just called one...*a fad.*

Trainers can tell who is serious about attaining their goals by their emotional response to these two criteria. If people haven't really made the decision to take action, they won't follow through on either or all of learning about 1) Whole-foods, 2) Functional-foods and 3) Certain dietary supplements at certain times or they refuse to acknowledge what their body composition means or they won't go get their blood chemistry panel done...they don't want to know. In these cases, the person has made the decision to *talk about* change or consider talking to an expert, but hasn't made the decision to take action themselves...a very fine distinction, but a very important one from the standpoint of whether or not a person is ready to be helped...*ready to change* in order to get different results.

So, in relation to the *Catch-22*, there's a phenomena I've consistently noticed over the years. If people have enough nutrition density (vitamins, minerals, enzymes, protein, fiber, good fats, etc.), in their diet, beginning early in life, they tend to crave nutritiously dense foods and the process continues on that path (they have established a standard of what being nourished looks and feels like). The side-affect of being well nourished (I'm talking about the brain being nourished, not the ego reacting and saying it has enough without knowing) is that people crave nutritious foods and do not crave S.A.D.C.R.A.P., junk-food, sugary drinks, excessive coffees, alcohol or none of that...*they are moderate in their choices.* People who are well-nourished tend to have more emotional stability and make decisions with the part of the brain known as the pre-frontal cortex of the brain...the part that makes rational decisions, considers options, recognizes love, attention and affection and enables good reasoning ability. People who are well-nourished are able to think about their thoughts, consider the options and make decisions based on fueling the body...[their hands grab healthy snacks]. They enjoy talking about nutrition and don't negate the power of nutrition nor behave as if they have heard enough...they're always looking for ways to improve. They want the edge and don't leave any stone unturned. Their choices are well thought out and not based on emotional whims... *their hands pay for and grab high nutritionally-dense foods and supplements.*

I've also consistently noticed over the years that the people whose diets are lacking nutrition density (vitamins, minerals, enzymes, protein, fiber, good fats, etc.), tend to crave sugary, fast energy, S.A.D.C.R.A.P., desserts, alcohol, rich coffee drinks, desserts and *THAT* process continues on that path. The side-affect of being poorly nourished (I'm talking about the brain being poorly nourished, not the ego reacting and saying it has enough without knowing) is that people tend to crave low nutrition density foods, mostly excluding nutritious food, even detesting it and insisting that nutritious food makes them sick (there's a clear reason for this). People in this scenario tend to say things like, *"I can't eat just one"* or *"Everything I eat goes to my butt"* and so on. The poorly nourished person tends to be the one who has less emotional stability, more of a compulsive aspect to food going out of their way to make poor choices in relation to their goals...the poorly nourished brain isn't fueled enough for the pre-frontal cortex to function properly and operates more out of the emotional center of the brain also known as the limbic system. When people are operating out of emotions they aren't as able to monitor their own thoughts, motives, motivations or think beyond simply getting sugar or other stimulants into the brain as soon as possible...*their hands pay for and grab poor nutrition food, yet withhold the B.N.B.B.s seemingly on-purpose.*

Poorly nourished people don't want to hear about nutrition, negate the benefits of dietary supplements and insist nutrition isn't the answer while complaining they can't control their emotions or impulses to eat a whole cake or drink a whole bottle of wine. Malnourished people will spend ten bucks a day on poor nutrition stuff but complain that the same ten dollars is too much for supplements...*a noticeable side effect of a malnourished brain:* The malnourished brain is always on the lookout for the next quick fix and rationalizes these decisions. An explanation that the malnourished person is always on the lookout for the next quick fix is because the brain doesn't store energy in it like the muscles and liver do...the brain uses about 25% of the body's fuel, but doesn't store a significant amount in itself...when the brain doesn't have enough nutrition to fuel the pre-frontal cortex it's kind of reduces energy output from higher thinking and rationalizing to lower level functioning of emotionally driven behavior to simply keep the brain fueled on sugar, salt, bad fats and caffeine (the hands grab low nutrition food and drinks).

As long as this process goes uninterrupted, the person keeps seeking fast-energy junk foods (which builds fat via insulin resistance) and avoids healthier, slow-energy choices (which facilitate burning fat for energy via insulin sensitivity). The more a person gives into junk food, the less attractive healthy foods which burn fat seem, since at the autonomic level, as the brain is primarily focused on keeping itself functioning because the brain keeps the rest of the body going! In other words, the more you eat junk food the more the brain wants junk food and is "turned off" by nutrient-dense foods...it's a matter of nutritional focus that happens at the unconscious level, until you consciously take the B.N.B.B.s on a daily basis to make up for the nutritional deficit.

The under-nourished brain doesn't recognize its under-nourished, but the [nourished brain recognizes that IT WAS undernourished, once it has a track-record of adequate nourishment]. Knowing that people want to start seeing and feeling results from their fat burning program as soon as possible, while learning to do resistance-training, cardiovascular-training and getting nutrition density into the diet, is it wise to pile on learning to cook nutritious food too? Some would argue, …*"Yes,"* but again, over forty years of personal experience with nutrition, I've seen the number one deterrent for the majority of the population is *"What do I eat?"* and *"I don't have the energy to cook or decide what to eat."*

By the time people learn to shop and cook (which they ultimately will do), they have already dropped out of their program from malnutrition. I haven't seen a person who insists knowing how to shop is the key to their fat-loss. But I do see people who make sure they get their supplements on a daily basis have the energy, mental clarity and focus to take a sincere interest in learning about food and cooking. For the person who isn't craving healthy food, yet and doesn't have their emotions lined up for success, the first things out of their mouth when you tell them what will help them the most is, *"I don't like that"*....duh! until they get enough nutrition density into their brain and body they don't want to eat nutritious food! *A Catch-22!*

A person can insist they don't like certain foods, but to simply supplement the diet with dietary supplements, regardless of what they "think" their taste is gives them the full benefit advantage of optimal nutrition without the nutritional gaps associated with picky-eating or lack of nutritional or cooking knowledge...*it eliminates the learning curve the first day.* If a person is all wrapped up in their emotional beliefs that supplements don't do anything then they're at a disadvantage from the get-go since it's really a waste of time to attempt to convince a person of something that they are emotionally attached to, even when it puts them at a *dis*-advantage..*irrational beliefs* or would otherwise be good for their health. A great example of the person who says they want help, but then won't do what they need to do! If a person is undernourished, the part of the brain that comprehends information about nutrition isn't functioning enough to fully consider the information.

I also noticed over these thirty years that the people who say they "believe" in supplements and simply start on a sensible supplementation program, they crave healthy foods and usually call me saying, *"You can't believe what happened"*, and then go on to tell me how they did everything I said to do and they're getting amazing results...*just like that*. The difference being that people who focus, *FIRST*, on getting their nutrition density up, by filling in their nutritional gaps, get faster results, find it easy to stick to their program, have very little if any cravings (cravings indicate malnutrition) and are constantly telling me how thankful they are to know me. The people who say, *"I'll do the nutrition stuff once I'm in shape"* last about three months before they are too tired, lose motivation, getting bored, get injured and figure they aren't going to be able to reach their goals. Nine months later they reset their New Year's Resolutions and it starts over, but they've gained another 5-10 pounds of fat, or more.

A Catch-22 is that the undernourished brain doesn't crave nutrition and without enough nutrition, will-power, motivation and emotional-stability are not achieved. A lot of trainers will accept clients who insist they know better when it comes to nutrition, but you have to remember that trainers get paid whether you follow through or not. Trainers can't turn away clients who don't follow through, they simply know the client will wonder why other clients are getting faster and better results and the ones who won't do the nutrition stuff from the start will flake-out in three months anyway...they won't do what the trainer says to do, then they insist they don't "get" why they aren't getting results (even though they are told that would happen) and then, since after three months they're getting minimal results they can't justify the cost of a personal training...duh? Truthfully, I believe that most people who seek personal training think that people get amazing results because they *hired* the trainer, rather than because of the clients who simply take the suggestions of the trainer and consistently follow through!

Chapter conclusion:

The Catch-22 of sustainable fat-loss is that the body requires high nutrient density (what I refer to as the B.N.B.B.s) to maintain an optimal emotional state, but malnourished people don't "feel" like getting enough nutrition density because a symptom of lack of B.N.B.B.s is a craving for S.A.D.C.R.A.P. *and an aversion to nutrition density*. "Feeling like" doing the correct action to achive your goals is based on adequate nutrition in your brain, *for you*. Lack of nutrition and you don't "feel like" doing it. To interrupt this cycle, you have to force yourself (get over the hump), to get nutrition density. Certain dietary supplements at key times are the easiest, most sensible and most cost-effective means of assuring you're getting a [consistent] amount of the B.N.B.B.s on a daily basis (cheaper than food). Inconsistent nutrition density is the crux of all fat-loss efforts.

Lack of nutrition density consistency is the single greatest factor to reaching, sustaining or missing out on your fat-loss goals, especially related to the emotional states related to fat-loss. In the decades of my professional experience, no other factor has seemed to have greater significance to seemingly effortless progress than simply getting enough B.N.B.B.s on a daily basis. It's that simple. Without adequate nutritional density, emotional stability is unlikely. People who are under nourished and seem to have an aversion to nutrition continue to struggle to burn fat and keep it off.

Whether you clean up the emotions first or get the nutrition consistently doesn't matter, as long as you do both. Nutrition density for fat-loss means: 1) Whole-foods, 2) Functional-foods and 3) Certain kinds of dietary supplements at key times (B.N.B.B.s). A Catch-22 of fat-loss is that cardiovascular exercise (cycling, rowing, running, walking, swimming), will burn fat, but without adequate nutrition (1) Whole-foods, 2) Functional-foods and 3) Certain dietary supplements at certain times), you'll unfortunately be unable to retain your lean mass...the only way to know if you're getting enough nutrition to retain your lean mass is through monitoring your body composition the first of each month (30-day average). But without certain supplements at the correct times, by the time you realize you're deficient, you've already hit a plateau in progress, regardless how much you increase your exercise intensity, frequency or duration.

Without supplementation, the more you exercise the more lean mass you'll lose. Without proper supplementation, you're unwittingly wasting time, energy and money. A lot of people who seem malnourished seem to enjoy arguing about nutrition.

An argumentative attitude is common with undernourishment, especially extra B vitamins. (its actually more simple to put the B.N.B.B,s in your body than to argue about them). But, the science doesn't lie. You can debate whether food has enough nutrition all you want. The scientific way to know is whether or not you're retaining and gaining lean mass, bone density and experiencing improvements in your blood chemistry numbers. A person who isn't nourished, will struggle to get their blood chemistry numbers in the healthy zone, regardless how healthy they insist they eat or how much nutrition they argue is in whatever food they choose. Body composition is a great indicator when people insist they are getting enough nutrition from food alone.

Activation of the "thinking"/cognitive/goal-achieving part of the brain and de-emphasis, on the abnormally high, emotional/instant-gratification aspect of the brain requires adequate nutrition density. It's as simple as people getting grouchy, angry and emotional when their blood sugar gets low. *We're all aware of this.* It's just that many people are in this state chronically, and not knowing that what resolves the phenomena is the B.N.B.B.s. So far, I don't know of any medical test that measures this [process] of how much B.N.B.B.s a person has in their frontal-brain and how it corresponds to behaviors. But, we can clearly see the behaviors and hear the language patterns, especially when comparing the before and after behavioral improvements from consuming and having enough B.N.B.B.s. Just like a lot of mental processes, deductive-reasoning, paying attention and comparing behaviors over the long haul shows the connection between fat-loss and consistent, proper consumption of the B.N.B.B.s. Its like night and day.

"90% of my experiences are described in this book. I think your books are great! I'm sure I was extremely under-nourished, highly malnourished. I lose weight then gain it back. I can't stand eating vegetables, unless they're cooked. I tried "cleansing", the Keto diet and the candida cleanse. I've gotten heavier and heavier, weaker and weaker. I don't want to be here any more. Can you give me a hand? I look forward to the day I crave vegetables. I want to lose 50 pounds of fat, get my body composition down to 15% and get my strength & health back and start doing fitness events after I burn off the fat."

T.M. Montana, March 2018

Chapter Eight

How Fast Is Fast?

For the most part, what people who hire a trainer say they are looking for is fast results (faster than they would get on their own). As discussed earlier, most people are willing to hurt their health if they think they can get the miracle-fix for the side-affects of consistent, poor lifestyle choices. I've had clients who took amphetamines to lose "weight" only to have their hearts damaged, clients who literally starve themselves and everything in-between.

Back in the 1970's and even into the 80's it was considered unhealthy to lose more than about two pounds a week. That's partly because, at that time much of what was considered medical weight loss revolved around doctor-supervised fasting...meaning dangerously low-calorie diets that aren't healthy in any way, *yet "medically-supervised".*

Under those circumstances, before most people knew about concepts like body composition and gaining lean mass while burning fat, bone density and blood chemistry labs to measure underlying health, the best they knew to do was force a starvation effect by drastically reducing calories at any cost to the health (the myth of calories-in, calories-out). The supervision part was just to discontinue the diet once side effects and harm to the health started showing up.

Today, some people including some medical practitioners still promote "calorie reduction" as healthy and relevant...*"calories-in, calories-out".* To review, inadequate calorie consumption results in the body using all the healthy tissue (lean mass) for energy and rationing or preserving body-fat in a sort of starvation effect. (On calorie reduction diets, the fat is the last thing to go, if at all, yet they stimulate significant gain of fat following the conclusion of the diet).

To compound the nutrition density problem, the less calories you eat, the less nutrition density you're getting...the more you restrict calories to lose weight the more you're compounding the problem of excess body-fat...you're going backwards.

So, any change in what the scale says on a calorie reduction program is mostly the healthy tissue loss and cannot necessarily be trusted. The amount of calories your body requires is based on how active you are, how healthy you are, how much body-fat you have, how much lean mass you have and a host of other factors related to where you are the day you begin your program.

The first of each month, you should recalculate your body composition, your resting heart rate and caloric requirements for the next month. If you don't do this process, its similar to getting in your car to travel to your destination, but then taking random streets going in all different directions, but insisting you're on your way and running out of gas before you get there.

Nutrition density (the amount of nutrition) you get each day is a higher priority (more important) than calories themselves. In other words, whether your calories are correct or not, if your nutrition is too low you won't get the intended fat-loss effects. Nutrition density is the primary facilitator of fat-loss, for many reasons. People that figure this out early get much more satisfying results, whether they believed it or not. I know this to be the case because I keep track of the body composition of my clients and track the results as well as the differences in progress between the people who apply the nutrition parts from the beginning and the ones who skip them, all things being equal.

The people who apply the nutrition are amazed how effective their program is while [the ones who avoid nutrition tend to gain more fat and lose lean mass] the more progress they make in their program. That's right, since their body goes into a kind of starvation-mode and rationing nutritional resources, their body gains fat and loses lean mass.

Ideally, you want to focus on feeding/fueling the lean mass and utilize certain exercise strategies to burn the fat. This is a difference between a novice trainer and an experienced one. Novice trainers generally encourage starving the body since they're more concerned about short-term appearances than long-term health. Without health, any body-fat lost from starving will return and then some.

With these factors in mind, I've found some averages. People who don't apply the nutrition parts to their exercise program will lose and gain about a pound and a half, bouncing back and forth every other week. Down one week, up the next but no practical, consistent results. If a person is hit-and-miss with their nutrition (meaning they skip the B.N.B.B,s), they'll lose a little bit more, but have greater swings in body weight, with little improvement in body composition.

The people who apply nutrition the way I described earlier as a complete nutrition program with 1) Whole-foods, 2) Functional-foods and 3) Certain dietary supplements at specific times, will burn between 12 and 20 pounds every month until they reach their goal and then effortlessly maintain it while improving all of their health markers.

So, to me, healthy, fast fat-loss means about 12 to 20 pounds of fat-loss, *per month*. If someone isn't burning that much fat I know that either their resistance training isn't designed or being carried out correctly, their cardiovascular exercise is either designed or carried out incorrectly or they don't know what to do nutritionally...sometimes it's a combination of two or three altogether. Skipping or substituting the B.N.B.B.s, being the most commom mistake.

Again, we're talking about knowing what the 12 to 20 pounds is by measuring body composition...not the scale alone. Without body composition measurements you could lose 12 to 20 pounds of lean mass and at the same time had either no reduction in fat or having gained even more fat. This is common and the reason body composition is so important. One client I had at Gold's Gym, Seattle avoided my nutrition suggestions as well as body composition testing, insisting he was, "*...working out hard enough to reach his goals*," (he hired me but knew better than me). When he agreed to being checked, after months of consistent workouts, he had gained 15 pounds of fat and lost 15 pounds of lean mass.

The most common mistake I've seen is when people insist they are doing a program the way it was demonstrated to them, but when I check it they are convinced they are doing what they were shown, but they aren't doing it correctly at all.

When I first started working out, my personal trainer (Tracy) designed a program for me, I did it exactly as she showed me and I got amazing results.

Being unable to comprehend what's being shown or taught is a side effect of malnutrition and emotional interferences. Without adequate nutrition in the brain, its near impossible to learn, let alone remember and recall...that's why it's emphasized for school children to eat breakfast.

Without the B.N.b.B.s on board, the brain can't retain the very information that could save it's life.

Today, I screen out potential clients, by which ones call me to get started on the B.N.B.B.s. If someone doesn't start off with a solid nutrition program I simply am not going to invest the time in it. The person who calls me to get their B.N.B.B.s squared away are the ones that get my time and expertise. And they're the ones which will get the best results the first month, which results in greater referrals of new clients.

If someone doesn't start with the B.N.B.B.s then I know they won't get results and I won't get any referrals from them.

Chapter conclusion:

If you're losing less than 12-20 pounds of fat per month, something is "off"...*ask me for help.*

"It was the first time my stomach problems went away and I felt so good the next morning I ran four miles." S.W., West Seattle, WA

Chapter Nine

Four Influences

There are four main influences that are intertwined in existence (physical, mental, emotional & spiritual). All four have equal influence over the others, but when any lack attention or any are given free reign, imbalance over the other influences occurs.

When the emotions are allowed to either take precedence over the other influences or are not managed adequately they certainly affect and influence the other three influences. Whatever you focus on grows. We can think of examples where someone focuses on their physical health, but lack mental clarity. Or someone who focuses on the spiritual aspects but ignores their physical well-being.

Its common sense that if you don't pay some attention to each area some, then imbalance occurs.

For the sake of the context of fat-loss, the emotions tend to be the greatest inhibitor of the physical and mental aspects of fat-loss when simply doing the workouts and nutrition doesn't seem consistently achievable. This effect primarily comes from mismanagement of emotional-content which leads to excessive physical and mental energy being used to prevent feeling and ultimately affects the spirit of the individual.

Chapter conclusion:

The physical, mental, emotional and spiritual aspects of life are all important and deserve mutual attention and development. The most common interrupter of sustainable, healthy fat-loss is related to the emotions related to the past, influencing the other three...*letting the emotions run you, versus experiencing in the moment and then moving on.*

"I can honestly say Sov has radically changed my life."
L.R., Blillings, MT

Chapter Ten

Body As A Vehicle For Emotions

In my experiences, the body is a dynamic, fluid, ever-changing entity that I think we've only seen the surface of what its capable of, under *the right conditions*. I've seen more miracles in relation to health and well-being than many might believe possible. What I'm referring to is that *change occurs in an instant,* when hope or prognosis for improvement was unexpected.

That the body is by design a flexible, changeable form mirrors the potential of the body and is a strength, but free-will and the influence of the mind over the body permits interference by the mind and emotions. Did you get that? We have free will and our experiences are enhanced by our ability to think what we want. We also can enrich each experience by allowing the emotions to come and go. We have the innate potential to be healthy, but we can interfere in our own well-being with how we use mind and emotions.

When I started out as a massage practitioner, I intended to primarily work with athletes. In massage school I saw the amazing metamorphosis that occurs when people simply let go the emotional-content of the past. Often, physical symptoms were rooted in emotional-content "stored or contained" within the body. As a clinical massage practitioner doing mainly injury treatments for auto accidents, on-the-job injuries, sports injuries and so on, I observed similar patterns. Regardless of the injury, once the emotions related to the injury or what lead up to the injury, (trauma) are released, change occurred in an instant, even defying the accepted standards of healing time. Years later, as a clinical hypnotist, the same patterns emerged. Regardless of what a person was asking for help for, mostly the symptoms came down to clearing up and gaining closure on past events and misunderstanding. The content being related to one-time events and sometimes situations that went on for some time.

What I have found is that if the situation is approached respectably and almost in a sacred fashion, once the emotional-content is cleared up, *change occurs in an instant.* An example would be if a person has an unexplainable pain in their shoulder that refers down their arm. If done with sufficient attention, massaging the arm and the person releases the emotion related to the pain and suddenly the problem is gone. Sometimes people have conscious recall of the original stressor (cntent) and sometimes they don't. Not every problem is emotion-based, even if there is an emotional component. Some people simply don't retain emotions let alone suppress them to the point where it's affecting their physical health.

How does storing of emotions happen?

When we experience stress or anxiety and the breathing changes to a holding the breath or reducing the number of breaths, whatever the stressor that is being perceived at the time gets more or less locked into the body, like glue. Each person tends to store and hold stress in a different part of the body individual to them, but there are common patterns. Holding the breath kind of glues/adheres emotional-content into the tissues. Deep breathing helps release the glue effect, releasing emotional-content from the tissues.

People who tend to not retain emotions think, *"Why would you do that?!"*

In my experiences, for lack of better explanation, it's as though when people have stress, how they deal with it is to put it somewhere (compartmentalize the stress) (put it somewhere safe until it can be fully comprehended, sorted and coped with, at a later time) the same we do with any project we're working on.

The problem seems to arise when we don't go back and visit or process the experience after the initial stress is over, either because we forget or because it involved psychological trauma that we would rather not have to deal with. In the military, 'revisiting' stress is referred to as "de-briefing". De-briefing is a way to help people process and understand what occurred, when they were too close to comprehend the big picture, as it was occurring.

Sometimes people either weren't prepared or weren't anticipating what they experienced, or they don't even have a frame of reference to comprehend what they experienced. In these cases, people tend to unconsciously stuff the experience away (somewhere in the body or mind) while they deal with the situation at hand. But this gives the benefit of the doubt that the person had the coping skills, maturity and perspective to deal with what they experienced.

Everyone has a different and varying level of coping with stress. Even soldiers who go through training aren't equipped to fully process what they experience as they experience it. If you picture combat (a firefight where multiple shooters are shooting at each other [high intensity and frequency]) and there simply isn't time to process stuff quickly enough because they have to act, without thought in order to stay alive and protect each other. In other words, telling people they'll see death and lots of injuries isn't enough to prepare every person for death and lots of injury.

For children who go through stress, often they live through experiences that even adults shouldn't have to or aren't skilled to cope with. If the stress happens once it might be intense, but if it occurs more than once over time, then it's a chronic stress, which affects the mind, emotions and personality in different ways. Sometimes its just a matter of a person having string feelings that they don't know what to do with at the time.

In other cases, a trauma might happen so intensely and so quickly that the mind can't keep up with what's happening regardless of one's age, maturity or coping ability. I helped a few clients who had been in high speed, head-on collisions in their automobile. Their body goes through all the trauma, but they don't necessarily consciously know everything that happened, since it was a blur. I experienced the same thing during a helicopter crash. So much went on so fast that I couldn't consciously remember all of it, but it still affected my body and I had bruises showing up days later, in areas which I wasn't conscious of ever being hit.

And then I had some clients who had really intense experiences early on, which lead to a seeming pattern of being accident prone, where they are so traumatized they seem to go from one trauma to the next and it seems to affect their ability to make good decisions in health and relationships and their safety, in general. Incorporating balance exercises into the workout routine help people integrate the past, even if they aren't consciously aware of the stress.

There's a wide range of what can happen to lead to emotional pain and *dis*-associative patterns, but the common denominator is that even though emotions are intangible (non-physical), they can directly affect the tangible (physical) well-being (like the mind to the brain) or the emotions on body compsotion levels and ultimately the hormones and other systems of the body. Not everyone is adept at understanding what's occurring let alone sorting it all out, but exercise and thorough nutrition done with guidance and consistency can facilitate the expression and integration of past experiences.

Chapter conclusion:

When the physical body is used to contain the emotions related to stress or trauma, one net result is increased body-fat. The longer the stress is contained or the more stress that is contained, the relative mass of the body (fat) increases exponentially.

"I have gotten better results in the last week and a half, more muscle...more definition, than I have in the last two years...I have learned from you that to get great results you have to give your body time to recover." S.F., Seattle, WA

Chapter Eleven

Healthy Relationships

Relationships are a very important factor in relation to success or difficulty with any fat-loss program. Healthy, supportive relationships can accelerate success in any context or endeavors. The most common difficulty trainers see with their clients is when the client is in relationship with someone whom they had common (unhealthy) activity and eating habits with when they met, but then one person wants to get healthy and move on to a fitness-lifestyle and their spouse doesn't have any intention or motivation to do so.

Ultimately, we're talking about varying degrees of co-dependency here. There's entire books and twelve step programs available, based on the concept of helping people recover from co-dependency. In short, one aspect of how it relates here is when one half of a couple cannot move on with their life because the second half isn't ready to improve, too!

A most common way this shows up (in the fat-loss context) is when the mom of the family usually does all the cooking for the family and eats whatever else everyone wanted cooked...the problem arises when mom begins a fat-loss program and doesn't want to cook the unhealthy meals anymore, but the family doesn't want to eat the healthy food nor cook their own meals (the co-dependency aspect is that mom is more concerned with everyone else's "feelings" about cooking for themselves than she places importance on her own health and progress) or blames other family members for why they can't adhere to their program.

When a person is too concerned or feels responsible with what another person *feels*, to the neglect of their own health, they're operating out of co-dependency. This isn't to be mistaken for concern for another's feelings, it's just that taken too far, either one or both people lose enough sight of themselves that they aren't operating in their own best interests anymore.

A second condition trainers and health professionals see in their practice is sabotage by another. An extreme case would be someone providing alcohol for an alcoholic (enabling). A less extreme example would be if one spouse knows their spouse is on a fat-loss program, but then continues to offer S.A.D.C.R.A.P. to them as if they don't know how challenging it can be to eat healthy anyway...they don't want the person to suffer the perception of missing out on consuming the stuff that is hurting them, so they enable/permit the person to keep doing behaviors that hurt them...in the guise of love. In other words, they mistake allowing/permitting hurtful behavior as being loving...versus being loving as preventing further self-harm.

I recall a story about a man in his thirties who was obese and diabetic. He already had both legs amputated, due to complications of high blood sugar/diabtes, but didn't make any changes to his lifestyle. Ultimately, he went to the hospital with his mom as his blood sugar was dangerously high. His mother was screaming at the medical staff to, *"...do something!!!"*, as she insisted they weren't helping him enough. When the staff returned to the room, they could see that the man's mother had run out to a well-known burger place and was feeding her son burgers, fries and shakes, screaming that the staff wasn't doing enough to help him. He didn't make it out of the hospital alive.

If one half the couple is ready to get healthy and live a lean lifestyle and the other half is satisfied indulging in S.A.D.C.R.A.P. it's going to take some pretty determined self-discipline to follow through with the constant temptation, exposure and influence. Or, if one half of a couple is ready to start a program but the other half has insecurity issues going on and instead of being supportive and joining in, the indirectly discourage, dismiss and undermine their partner's attempts.

If the partner who isn't intending to get healthy feels like they are being abandoned its very common for them to passive-aggressively interfere in hopes of derailing the other's good intentions. The severity of the interference depends on the personality and dynamics of the individuals. It's not uncommon for people to start working out and get a personal trainer as a statement of their individuality, when they are ready to move on from a relationship or at least declare their independence from being codependent.

But, if you're the half of the couple who is getting fit and you want to reassure your spouse, it will go a long way to let them know how important this is to you and that you're still here with them, that you're going to improve some things, but you still love them and you'll be there for them in a newer, better version. You can't go wrong with pouring on the pre-emptive reassurance.

Simply repeating this process can give your spouse space to observe and contemplate their own health and state and if you're both committed to each other, once you are getting good results, they'll likely join you. Invite them to join you. Even when people are stuck and overwhelmed, there's usually a part that wants to improve and be free of the prison of fat and ill health. It's just that often one person in a couple is better at change and motivation than the other. Fat-loss always works better if both halves of the couple do it together or you at least have a buddy to do it with. This is one of the things I screen potential clients for.

If you do have an insecure, sabotaging-type partner, you've got your work cut out for you, since you'll be maintaining you own emotional status as well as theirs (co-dependency), which is neither healthy, nor sustainable. In order to succeed, you'll have to prioritize your own progress. That doesn't mean abandon your spouse, it means find ways to maintain the bond, but get very clear and disciplined about your own exercise and nutrition practices. There has to be certain hours of the day when you take care of yourself, without interruption or interference.

Using others (or caring for others) as a reason why you can't exercise and get your nutrition is a scapegoat.

If you have children and they're mature enough to make some meals too, then simply involve them in the changes you're doing and they'll likely take it and run with it. Kids love getting healthy and they love talking about S.A.D.C.R.A.P. If you family is dependent on S.A.D.C.R.A.P. and doesn't want healthy food, then take your own B.N.B.B.s in front of them. Taking supplement, in front of someone, is the most efficient way to help them get started. Don't try to convince them, just let them see you taking them. The more malnourished they are the longer it may take for them to catch on, but once again, as you stick to your program they'll see the changes and those inclined to get healthy anyway, will ask you to teach them. It's better to clear all the junk food out of the house, but if your family isn't participating it might make more sense to let them have their junk food as long as you don't consume it at all. People who are addicted to S.A.D.C.R.A.P. are going to buy it again anyway after throwing it out, which indicates malnutrition and lack of B.N.B.B.s in the brain.

Circle of influence:

A big part of success in any context is the people in your circle of influence. There's a saying that each person's income will be the average of the five people they socialize with the most. I've found it to be true in relation to health and fitness too...that each person will be as fit and healthy as the average of the five people they socialize with.

An important distinction here is that the idea is not to abandon your friends and family, although after you hear their comments about you getting healthy you might consider it! What I'm talking about is expanding your circle of influence. By simply making a few acquaintances who have similar goals, you'll really get a lighter feeling about what you're accomplishing.

If you're hesitant or introverted, the easiest thing to do is to begin signing up and participating in charity fun-run/walks. There are literally thousands of these fun runs around the country every year. The signup fee is low, you usually get a t-shirt and often there's prizes. The point is being "around" people with similar interests and values. There's usually fun-runs for every holiday and every organization you can think of and nobody cares if you walk the whole way or run. Start out with 5ks (about three miles).

You can also do a web search for clubs in your area for walking, cycling, running, etc., for groups that meet on a regular basis. People in these groups are usually very welcoming and love having new, positive members. From there, you'll meet people you get along with and probably do other activities too. The possibilities are endless and you can post pictures of yourself at the events on your social website, finding people you already know who you didn't know you had this in common with.

Not everyone is supposed to get along with everyone, it's just not common for it to happen that way. When there isn't a connection simply move on and meet more people.

Chapter conclusion:

There are co-dependency groups in every state and internationally. If relationship seems to prevent or interfere in your efforts, you can seek free help through Codependents Anonymous.

http://coda.org/

The primary book used by Codependents Anonymous is available through Amazon, entitled *Co-Dependents Anonymous.*

"...what you do makes people live longer...you give people more life...it's hard to quantify that...it's not like buying a car, you extend a person's life whether its five days or five years." B.D., Seattle, WA

Chapter Twelve

Notice Emotional Self-Tricks

Self-tricks are related to giving yourself permission or a "hall-pass" to do something that you know [isn't] in alignment with your goals, then rationalizing or minimizing that you did it. Skipping "just one workout" or "having one piece of cake" or going to a bar to have "just one drink" are examples of self-tricks. Sometimes its referred to as falling-off-the-wagon, but regardless of what you call it, it relates to thinking that since you've made some progress, you deserve a reward with a behavior that sabotages your goals. Falling-off-the-wagon is not a valid excuse, it involves and is the result of decisions, rooted in being inconsistent with the B.N.B.B.s. The more undernourished a person, the more often they insist they deserve a reward for behavior that is simply self-care and hygiene.

Now, I'm telling you as clearly as I can that if your B.N.B.B.s are up to snuff, it's unlikely you'll start telling yourself *"..a little bit of cake won't hurt...but I'll take the whole cake home just in case"*. The mind simply doesn't work that way when the nutrition level is high enough in the brain...it just doesn't happen. If you tell yourself you "think" your nutrition level is high enough, but still binge on S.A.D.C.R.A.P. then you're self-tricking yourself in that way. If you're eating S.A.D.C.R.A.P. your B.N.B.B.s aren't up to snuff even though your ego is ignoring the fact. If you're thinking about junk food or rewarding yourself with junk food, your B.N.B.B.s aren't up to snuff. So if you say something like, *"I fell off the wagon,"* you're really saying you consciously chose to skip the B.N.B.B.s knowing their would be negative consequences and did it anyway. I personally won't work with people like this. I simply don't have time to work with everyone that I'm getting requests from, so I limit my practice to those who follow my suggestions from the get-go and consistently follow through.

I've seen plenty of clients who get on their nutrition program, things are going wonderful for two or three months, then they tell themselves that they don't need the nutrition anymore and within weeks, one by one all the S.A.D.C.R.A.P. habits of sabotage are back in full force...and since their brain isn't in full cognitive function, they can't even remember why the cravings had gone away before...they can't connect the level of nutrition density to losing all cravings for junk food and in turn crave fruits and vegetables. Remember! The malnourished brain can't learn or remember or retain information it needs to keep itself healthy, especially when the brain clicked over into emotionally driven behaviors.

Then they get back on their nutrition program and all the cravings and self-indulgence recede and they're back to craving healthy whole-foods and feeling wonderful again.

Avoiding self-tricks simply means being cognitively aware enough to be honest with yourself and avoiding calling something other than what it is. The single greatest factor that prevents fooling yourself is getting enough 1) Whole-foods, 2) Functional-foods and 3) Certain kinds dietary supplements at specific times. The reason being that self-tricks are emotional-based decisions and is what happens when the brain doesn't have enough nutrition built up to fuel the non-emotional, thinking parts of the brain.

Almost like clockwork, as soon as people lower their nutritional standards and start skipping one or more of the three parts, they start rationalizing non-rational behaviors and then making excuses for why they had to have some junk food. As soon as they get the three parts back in order, they lose all attraction to junk food and can't believe the difference in how they feel and how they THINK.

Its predictable, common and I haven't seen any exceptions.

One of the most common ways this shows up is the client will insist they had to take care of a family member and couldn't find fresh fruits and vegetables or anywhere to workout. In reality, anyone can fit two hours into the day for food and exercise. There's simply no excuse unless you're physically incapable and the more stress you're under, the more you're taking care of others and so forth the more you need 1) Whole-foods 2) Functional-foods and 3) Certain supplements at certain times. The B.N.B.B.s buffer the effects of stress on the body.

Besides, you trainer has heard every excuse there is.

Chapter conclusion:

Self-tricks are when you give yourself permission to break the rules, tell little white lies, get off track and so forth, but minimize and fail to fully acknowledge the detrimental implications of them on your goals. The more malnourished you are, the less able you are to resist you own self talk/temptations. All those little self-tricks add up to a half-pound or two of fat gain per month (12-24 pounds, *or more* per year).

If you've been doing self-tricks and you don't know how to stop, 1) Acknowledge what's happening 2) Name it 3) Ask for help. Most likely you'll be reminded to focus on nutrition density...*force yourself to get nutritional density every day.*

Self-tricks are symptoms of lack of nutrition density in the diet, via lack of integrity to your goals and lack of will-power *(will-power is a function of the well- nourished brain).*

With the learning curve of selecting and preparing foods with high enough nutrition density to make up for the chronic deficit, most people will quit trying before they get enough nutrition density from food alone. It just doesn't happen.

"You have helped me so much...you made it fun...you have had the best affect of anyone...this really does work...with all the skills you bring to the sessions it would cost $500 an hour to go to separate people with all those skills." J.K., Seattle, WA

Chapter Thirteen

Feeling Versus Thinking:
Emotions, Gut-feelings, Intuition & Thinking

Every single day we have endless opportunities to improve ourselves and *create more choices* for ourselves and our family. Much of what personal trainers and health care providers do is help people realize more choices and opportunities...things that are available to us, but they may have been outside awareness, as of yet. There's a significant percentage, of the visits to personal trainers and medical care providers, which are related to lifestyle choices: *exercise and nutrition.* That's because in the absence of exercise and nutrition density, every system of the body suffers and progressively breaks down...*degenerative dis-ease.*

Honestly, the majority of the population doesn't want to change their lifestyle or habits even when it's a life or death situation (do me)...that's how we have 80% of the population carrying too much fat for their own health. Generally speaking, people get into a habit that isn't good for their health as a way to cope with a life stress, whether it was a single incident they are attempting to integrate or a longer-term or even chronic stress situation. A simple example would be someone stressed-out, so they begin smoking cigarettes, but even after the stress is over they continue to smoke. The choice to start smoking began out of relieving stress (dis-associating from the body), but the relief became a stressor in itself which hurts the health. I know, I know, some people smoke their whole lives and don't seem to have any health effects. I watched a guy on TV who had smoked over a million cigarettes in his life and had drank whiskey most of his adult life and he was in his nineties. His siblings were over a hundred years old. So, there are exceptions to everything, nature is funny that way and I leave room for miraculous variables, too.

For the most part, we know that carrying more than 20% body-fat has many short-term and long-term side effects. Most people who let their body-fat go for too long regret it. There certainly are the people while avoiding exercise and getting the B.N.B.B.s they insist they are doing what they want and are exercising their autonomy...*addicts do that!* In America, food and beverage is one of the most common ways people medicate themselves out of "feeling" the body they inhabit. When you hear people make comments like *"...food is my best friend"* you know they're in trouble, since they are depending on food as an emotional-crutch. Each food has a different affect on the brain. Some foods give a sense of euphoria and some cause a type of "checking-out" or *dis*-association...as if from an emotional and cognitive viewpoint, people learn to live [a distance from their physical body]. People who are carrying too much body-fat really aren't feeling what it's like to be grounded in their physical body. The evangelist-type fitness gurus get it, but you don't have to go that far. You can have it all to yourself and pay it forward selectively.

The main reason I keep repeating and use the 20% body composition as the standard to measure initial fat-loss success, is that the closer you get to 30% body composition is where all the *de*-generative *dis*-eases kick in (heart *dis*-ease, high blood pressure, high cholesterol, high blood sugar, respiratory problems, immune system problems, digestive problems, etc., etc.,). Once you're past 30% you're in the danger zone. Someone could have a BMI considered within normal limits, yet be at more than 20% body fat.

And then you have the people who insist being fat proves they love themselves and accept themselves as they are, so they consider themselves role models for others...big bones, family genetics, etc., (remember, even if you have big bones your body composition shouldn't be more than 20% unless you want to get seriously ill). When the body composition is more than 20% (for a sedentary person) it manipulates the hormones of the body and ultimately leads to *dis*-ease. These are cases of what we talked about earlier (perfecting the neurosis...finding a way to keep doing the unhealthy thing so well that no one could seem to have a rational argument about, it nor have an affect on it from the outside).

If you intend to participate in athletic or fitness events, your body composition needs to be between 10% and 20%.

One of the emotional-based variations to people who can't seem to successfully do exercise and nutrition is the contrary-attitude...the *"I'll do the opposite of what I pay you to teach me to do and you can't make me do it"* attitude. You know that saying, *"You're only fooling yourself"?*..it applies here.

There are some people who consistently seek out who they consider the coolest, hippest, most renowned expert to gain their input. They'll spend hours upon hours researching the next person they will insist they have to see, be on the waiting list for months, telling everyone they know that they're on the list with so-and-so, spend hours telling the expert their story and when the expert does whatever testing and assessments are within their scope of practice and finally gives their professional advice, the person begin arguing, insisting why the expert is in the dark, how the expert can't possibly be right, couldn't possible know them and couldn't possibly understand their situation and then proceeds to "fire" the latest professional...they go from professional to professional to professional doing the same thing over and over. If they go a couple months without getting a new one, they'll circle back around and make an appointment with one they already fired so they can do it again. Seriously!

Do you get what is missing in this scenario? *Simply doing exercise and nutrition…*avoidance…distraction…disassociation. Doing anyting, but the very habits that deliver you to your goals and away from what your compaints are.

Sometimes, these types are referred to as fickle, boomerangs or polar-responders...meaning they always do the opposite of what they are told to do by the people they beg to help them. A portion of the visits in every medical office go just like that. Many people are too under-nourished to take in the very information they need!

Short-term and long-term fat-loss results from [correct] exercise and nutrition...it's that simple.

Although in my practice I have it down to a science where people generally notice a difference in the way they feel and how their physique looks within three days of beginning, the people who have continued success simply learn the fundamentals and then learn a little bit more and refine what they do every three months get good results too. Unless someone just does the same things over and over even if they aren't getting results, they're likely to get some kind of results anyway. For me, any time I begin a new endeavor, I read at least five books on the topic and then find an industry expert and hire them to train me...makes sense, right? In that way you develop a base of the most popular and current-knowledge and information for whatever topic you're into.

"Yaaaay, but what I feel is..."

One of the sticking points for people (where they limit their own choices), is when they only use their mind one way for every situation. An example of this would be if someone has their body temperature taken and are told its 104°F degrees and they say, *"Yay, but I feel as though its 98.6°F degrees"...."...what I feel is"*.

Did you catch that? The fictional person avoided the truth or the seriousness of the matter by framing their response as though their "feeling" about the situation is more priority than the science of the matter. In these cases, people avoid using the word "think" and replace it with "feel" to avoid the responsibility of rational thought. I mean who would have the nerve to argue with what a person feels... right? -This is different than talking "about" feelings in relationships and so forth, where there has to be some easiness and informality within conversations or taking all angles of a situation into consideration.

This same dynamic happens with blood sugar levels (diabetes), blood pressure (cardiovascular *dis*-ease), cholesterol results, body-fat levels....even people who are in abusive relationships can get physically beaten up but reply with, *"Yes, he beats me, but I feel he's sweet."*

All of these examples are of people who are avoiding taking responsibility for their welfare by using language to distract themselves from the gravity of the situation. When you listen to your own language you become aware of how associated to your physical self you are. If you're using, *"Yay, but what I feel is...."* frequently, that could be a place where you're interrupting your own progress. I've never heard a person who was doing great with their exercise and nutrition program over-use "feel" in place of "think". Success with fat-loss is a thinking and doing thing, not a feeling thing. "Feel" implies rational thinking or doing, but is neither.

People double-deceive themselves if they then insist that the objection of answering everything with, *"Yay, but what I feel is..."* is about others saying their feelings aren't important (attempting distraction and displacement to avoid accountability). Your feelings are important. What is "off" is when people over use the idea of feelings as a way to avoid the responsibility and accountability of rational, self-care behavior, with rational thought.

In the context of speaking about you and your own body and health, when you use the word think, your mind literally transfers into thinking/rational mode and when you say "feel" there's often a disconnect that is related to being disassociated/checked-out from your physical body and what's good for it. The brain does this when its low on nutrition and its having to manipulate the person to focus on getting the blood sugar up for basic functioning of the body. The reason being is that when you say, *"Yay, but what I feel is...."* you're unconsciously avoiding the information and the person who spoke it right before you said it. It's a way to (seemingly politely) discredit and dismiss the facts you just received. As long as this disconnect is going on in your mind, you'll be unable to fully learn and retain the information you need to make decisions and consistently act on exercise & nutrition information you have insisted you want...the reason being is that to reach your goals, you'll have to exercise discipline (thinking) to do exercise and do nutrition even when you "feel like" you should take the day off or skip nutrition for the day. You have to exercise discipline to get your nutrition. Once you put enough in you'll develop a habit and really notice what it feels like to have too little nutrition, in your body and your body will give you direct feedback when you don't have enough nutrition for yourself. Without adequate nutrition (for you), the body isn't capable of providing feedback.

Discipline, motivation and will-power are FUNCTIONS of a highly nourished brain. When someone says they *"...went-off-the-wagon"* or *"...couldn't resist a food,"* what they are unconsciously saying is that they don't have enough nutrition density on board. The problem being that people who are malnourished aren't conscious they are malnourished...they simply notice the side effects of being malnourished...and don't know what the side effects mean or how it translates to behavior that prevents *"going off the wagon."*

Emotional richness:

Emotions are meant to be experienced to enrich each of life's experiences...and then released...holding onto emotions creates body-fat in most people.

Gut-feelings:

Gut-feelings are a phenomena, in which the nerve connection between the brain and the digestive system give a type of feedback which helps warn you if a situation isn't "right" whether it's because of caution, danger, safety, gathering more information before proceeding or simply being aware of your surroundings. Sometimes gut-feelings simply mean to need more information before making a decision. Gut-feelings tend to be rooted in information about your environment that is coming in through your sensory awareness organs. For example, you might be walking in the woods and the smell of a bear might be outside your conscious awareness, but your brain will certainly pick up on it and the gut feeling you get will come from information your nervous system has picked up even if you were distracted...the hair on your neck will stand up. You might sense danger, but be unaware of *why* or you might simply need more information to feel comfortable.

You shouldn't ignore gut-feelings. But in order to get the most of your gut-feelings, in terms of clarity and consistency (being able to trust your gut), you have to let go of a good portion of suppressed emotions from the past, since they can interfere with true, clear gut-feelings (suppressed emotions use up significant energy reserves making it near impossible to have clarity with gut-feelings). They're called gut-feelings, since the nervous system sends the impulses through the vagus nerve, into the digestive area where we can "digest" it.

When people tend to hold emotions in, they "cloud" gut-feelings. The people tend to say, *"...yay, but what I feel is,"* and what comes out of their mouth will likely not be in their own health best interest.

Intuition:

Intuition is a phenomena, in which we get information that seems to defy physical explanation. People who are spiritual or religious might say the message was from God or a guardian angel, others might call it their higher-power or even their higher-self. Intuitional information or hints defy our physical ability to get the information other than as a "knowing" or a hunch that turns out to be accurate. For example, if you have a goal and everyone you know is saying you won't make it or all the "facts" insist you're wrong, but an idea pops into your consciousness out of nowhere and you follow up on the information to find out that the idea, which defies logic turns out to be helpful.

Intuition often comes to us in the mind area although it can be sensed outside of us as well. You shouldn't ignore intuition. The more present and clear you are (the more work you've done to release old emotional baggage) the easier it will be to receive and be aware and respond to your intuition, since emotional baggage is a major distraction and consists of the past, while intuition is about the present and your future. Old emotional baggage distracts from having motivation and accomplishing things in the present because it exhausts all the systems of the body and mind.

When people tend to hold emotions in, they "cloud" intuition. The people tend to say, *"...yay, but what I feel is,"* and what comes out of their mouth will likely not be in their own health best interest. When so much energy is being used to utilize emotions to avoid exercise and nutrition, too much energy is being used to properly make use of intuition.

Thinking:

Again, emotions enhance experiences, gut-feelings protect us, intuition assists us and feelings enhance the experience of what we think about things, but in order to stick with your program, if you've had trouble sticking with a program in the past, thinking things through (a little bit) and then acting/doing/behaving will be your best friend. You can think about things all you want, but over-intellectualizing (mental-masturbation/mental-procrastination), won't change the reality that in order to take care of yourself, you'll need at least three hours of resistance training broken into one hour chunks each week and an hour of fat-burning, cardiovascular training broken into three sessions of twenty minutes each week (four hours: everyone has time for that).

All the research is in and exercise is good for and applies to everyone. Even people in wheel chairs and missing limbs exercise and participate in competitive sports.

If you're spending time trying to figure out how to burn fat without exercise and improving what you're putting in your body, you're simply wasting time. Sort out your thoughts from your emotions. During the times when you're doing these healthy activities, practice acknowledging your emotions, but practice setting your emotions aside for the time being...DO THE ACTIONS, acknowledge what you're feeling, but don't allow them to paralyze you into a fat existence.

If you're not sure what exactly to do, don't waste time pretending you do. Get up and go! Ask for help!

Chapter conclusion:

Residual emotions can interfere with gut-feelings, intuition and clear thinking. As you continue to increase your self-awareness, you'll be able to make better use of higher functioning aspects of yourself and life will seem easier.

"They need someone like you here. I think that's why you are getting so many clients." E.G., Seattle, WA

Chapter Fourteen

Forms Of Effective
& Ineffective Communication:

Venting, Gossiping, Processing, Sorting, De-briefing & Story Telling

As you know, from the list above, there's a few different kinds of communication and this list is not complete. Each type either builds a person up, improves self-esteem, enhances self-image and naturally increases energy or has the opposite effects.

A lot of people don't know when they are communicating to the outside world in ways that lowers their own self-esteem, decreases their self-image and interferes with their ability to re-charge naturally. A reason being that communication in general feels good, is satisfying and provides a sense connection to others. People who haven't naturally learned that some types of communication are harmful don't understand that the way they relate to others affects their own physical, mental, emotional and spiritual health & wellness. Carrying too much body-fat is one affect of relating and communicating with the self and others in ways that drains energy, depletes energy of self and unconsciously attempts to pull energy from other people via sympathy, attention and co-miserating.

Venting:

Venting is a way to let off steam and express what you think and feel you've experienced. Venting can be beneficial so that you don't let the stress build up which leads to a blow up! It's always better to discharge and cope with stress, as you go along, and exercise does this. People who vent in order to regain their composure generally do so and simply move on. Self-awareness comes into play here, as a person who isn't self-aware will either on purpose or unwittingly attempt to dominate conversations with venting and guiding the conversation back to themselves. Whether it's healthy, productive venting or "too much information" depends on the person's, intent (who is doing the venting).

One of the byproducts of unproductive, inappropriate venting is when the person does the venting to avoid improving themselves, using the vent session as a means to criticize others or even blame others for the emotional feeling they are having. People who tend to avoid or distract themselves from what they are feeling, coincidentally tend to lack healthy coping mechanisms. An example of healthy coping mechanisms is where the person stops trying to control other people or their responses and simply focuses on dealing with their own responses to outside stress. Unhealthy coping mechanisms would be when someone thinks that by talking about a situation they aren't happy with, over and over and over will somehow improve the situation, instead of exercising and building up their nutritional savings account, making themselves more resilient to stress.

How to know? A good standard is how many times you talk about the same situation. Three times is a general good standard to go by. Within three repetitions, you'll know if talking about the situation is improving it. Beyond three times, the person is generally feeding off the attention and sympathy of telling the story over and over. Retelling the story is an inadequate substitute for feeling like you're taking control and action of the situation.

If you find yourself retelling the same complaint, consider why you're doing it. It's usually a diversion from doing your own self-improvement work. You can use the same amount of energy to exercise and do some nutrition and ask the people you're talking to what's going on with them.

Gossiping:

Gossiping has similar depletion characteristics on the gossiper...*depletion and lowered self-esteem.*

There's a fine line between camaraderie and repeating stuff at others' disadvantage. If you think of a group of people who work together exchanging stories about what's going on at work, this can actually create a healthier work environment versus being suppressed and detached. The line is determined by your intent. If sensationalism and drama gives you a high, but you don't exercise and apply the three key principles of a complete nutrition program, you're likely gossiping to distract yourself from the work you need to do as well as to distract yourself from how poorly you feel about yourself. Gossip hurts both the person doing the gossiping as well as the person being gossiped about. Every time the gossip is repeated it hurts the person being talked about. Leave people to learn from their life instead of treating them like the learning process is unique to them. Everyone makes mistakes and learns at a different pace.

At first it might be a challenge to determine which category you're in, but it's easy to see who is fit, healthy, focused on the positive and putting more energy into improving their life versus those who avoid improving themselves and feed off negativity.

Another indicator is if the conversation is about a situation or about what happened to others or what another did. Some situations, especially things related to safety require being talked about so prevent injury of yourself and others. If safety is the issue, by all means, repeat the story and pass it on. By watching out for others, you'll improve your self-esteem and improve your self-image and your role in the world and subsequently build others up.

Processing:

Processing is a way to figure out, understand and integrate your experiences. When you go to a counselor, therapist, doctor or talk stuff over with your trainer, processing is part of this. An example of processing is when you have an experience and you either don't understand it, how it happened or are confused by some aspect of it, processing is what you're experiencing. The difference with processing is that the intent is to understand and then move on, versus repeating a story to gain attention or shed a negative light on others' misfortune.

Everyone has variations in their life experience, education, training and so forth. When we talk to others in order to solve problems or expand our choices processing helps.

Sorting:

Sorting is when you've had multiple experiences, often in such close proximity that it's difficult to separate the experiences and in such a case they influence you outside your awareness. If you've heard the saying, *"It's hard to tell where I start and where I end"* you get the idea. Confusion, inconsistency, emotional reactivity and mood shifts are examples of when some sorting is in order. A clear example would be where soldiers return from combat and they have had so many overlapping, stressful experiences that they have PTSD (too much sensory data in too short of time to integrate it). Other than combat, varying types of life experiences can have the same affects depending on each person's tolerance level, their ability to process and integrate experiences. What stresses one person might relax others.

Sorting is kind of like if you have a big pile of papers all mixed up versus having labeled files with everything in their right places. Information that is sorted allows you to make better use of the information and makes it more readily accessible, rather than having to look through everything every time you want to use a piece of it.

When things are sorted out, there's more emotional clarity, more ease and less energy being used for trying to keep things straight.

De-briefing:

De-briefing relates to talking about what just happened or happened in the past so that sorting, processing and integration can occur. There's a phenomena that occurs with the mind in that if people don't understand what happened, it's difficult to gain the lesson from the experience. If a person doesn't really understand what happened or how cause and affect have occurred, future experiences seem more stressful and adaptation to new experiences and stresses are more stressful...adaptation is difficult since the past isn't resolved.

De-briefing can be as simple as having someone tell you what happened in sequential order. *"First 'A' happened, then 'B' happened and that led to 'C'"*.

A common denominator among people who carry too much fat is that they insist they don't understand how they got that way...or they insist they know it all, but upon questioning, they can't explain it to others (lack of integration).

Story telling:

Story telling/teaching tales is when you have done enough processing, sorting, integrating (introspection; thinking about your thoughts) that you can take what you and others and have experienced and vicariously utilize those stories to help others you come across (paying it forward).

Story telling can seem like you're talking about yourself, but the difference is in the intent. To the listener, story-telling is different than gossip or venting because the listener ends up feeling motivated, inspired and looking forward to a brighter future. Story telling is a way to take what you have learned and enrich others' lives by introducing ideas, skills and various lessons that otherwise might stir up resistance, polar responses or opposing behaviors if presented as simple instructions. Essentially, story-telling takes the lemons you had in life and turns them into fresh lemonade for others enjoyment. Instruction is a left brain/analytical process, while story telling is a more creative/right brain process that allows others to understand without too much analysis occurring.

Story telling has the opposite effects on the teller as gossip and venting do. By telling stories that help lift others up, you naturally draw energy to you through good deed and freeing up your consciousness through enriching others. Gossip and venting tens to suck energy from people, but neglects natural energy from nature, whereas story telling makes both the listener and speaker feel better, which leads to a lighter emotional experience and that leads to motivation and being more active out in nature. Attempting to pull energy off people through sympathy is unnatural and imbalanced and leads to a greater deficit of physical, mental, emotional and spiritual energy.

The "body" as we refer to it gains energy through several means. The most basic is the result of the nutritional density (vitamins, minerals, etc.). In India, the physical body is called *Ana Maya Kosha*...translated to "the body that comes from food".

Adequate nutrition density builds up the physical, mental and emotional reserves. Each area builds up and benefits the other areas in synergistic fashions...*the sum is greater than the whole.* For example, physical nutrients benefit the emotional aspects which aren't tangible, yet affect the physical body. The more "emotional" reserve enhances physical activity through motivation, inspiration and goal attainment. When I speak of the B.N.B.B.s, these are some of the interacting processes people experience when they put the B.N.B.B.s in their body, on a daily basis. Any inconsistencies in putting the B.N.B.B.s in the body short changes the mental, emotional and ultimately the physical spirit of each person, not to be mistaken for the soul. When you have emotional reserve, your mental state is more clear and resilient and the intentions set by you are able to be carried out. When the physical body is lacking physical nutrition, it's very unlikely the person will maintain consistent forward momentum. I just never see it happen.

Chapter conclusions:

Listen to yourself. Often, there's ways we're communicating that feel good in the moment, but are actually interfering with us reaching our goals through depletion of energy. Be very clear about what you talk about to others, your intention for doing so and what you think you're gaining from doing so.

How you use or preserve your energy in communication carries over to accomplishing your goals. Any areas you conserve energy in communication will return in results from your workouts.

"It's a pleasure to meet someone so knowledgeable…my doctor knows a lot but he doesn't seem to know how it all fits together."
M.O., Seattle, WA

Chapter Fifteen

Qualities Of Being
Emotionally Present/Associated

In these next two chapters, I'm going to cover qualities of people who have become (often through intensive and consistent attention) emotionally present and positive enough to reach their goals and maintain their achievements, as well as people who have become (often unwittingly and without awareness) emotionally not present (*dis-associated*), and negative to the point of interfering in their own progress and unable to stick with a basic exercise and nutrition program (attitudes).

To a person who mostly entertains negative guests in their mind, they might spout off that they don't need anyone controlling their thoughts or getting inside their head. And my reply would be, *"Exactly! It takes too much energy to control other people...you have to control your own thoughts and get inside your own head,"* (having presence of mind).

No one is 100% positive 100% of the time. That's not reasonable and no one expects that. What we're talking about here is which side of the fence are you on 51% of the time and (when) you have an off-day or a bad experience, how do you respond, handle and manage yourself at those times? How well do you get yourself back on track?

In every endeavor, the people who are the very best and most successful aren't successful 100% of the time...they simply notice when they are off track, when they aren't getting the results they intend and then they simply adjust themselves to get back on course. Some of the most successful people in the world can be very emotional. They might really have an outburst when things don't go how they wanted, but the difference is that they [notice] what they are experiencing, [acknowledge] what they are experiencing (whether from the outside or inside), [name] it, [own] it and then get themselves back in a state of mind & emotion to continue making progress. In the beginning, it's more important to be aware and acknowledge what you're experiencing than to attempt changing without adequate awareness.

It's not at all unlike life, as we reach a new level of self-development, achievement or success to hand us an opportunity (challenge us) to re-focus, pull ourselves together and gear up for the next season of progress.

The people who are rooted in negativity or have a chip-on-their-shoulder will feel like they are having a harder time in life...things will seem harder and as if things take more energy. In reality, it's the allowing negativity to inhabit us that takes the energy away from endeavors, but negativity makes people feel as though negativity is the power position when in reality it's more like negativity "uses" us to funnel itself into the world and inhibits the success we so desire...*negativity pushes the thing we seek further into the future.*

Why negativity is exhausting and disempowering has partly to do with which hormones are being released in relation to the emotions...positivity stimulates healing and soothing hormones like testosterone, serotonin and dopamine, while negativity stimulates the stress hormones cortisol, adrenaline and norepinephrine, which literally breakdown and depress the body and mind (when released chronically). Gratitude, peace, joy, hope, faith and love decrease/buffer stress hormones while anger, anxiety, depression, resentment, regret, self-pity, frustration, worry and hopelessness increase/stimulate stress hormones.

In my lifetime, I started watching people's attitudes and the way they think and talk long before I ever became a trainer (as a little kid). Part of the reason was that I grew up very impoverished, but I was intensely curious about the differences between people who seemed to have an abundant seemingly "easy" life and the people who had an impoverished "hard" life. Ultimately, what I have seen so far is that "attitude" and perception are a couple of the greatest factors that determine what kind of a life a person has. I observed people who lived nearly next door to each other, one family in poverty and having one unfortunate event after another, while the other family (often extended family of the first family) have success and good luck one after the other.

In other words, beyond the external "conditions" or rational reasons why each person is living in or insists are the reasons why their life is so hard, what determines how their life turns out (regardless of how they started out) is based on their attitudes and perceptions and the meaning they make about their conditions, their role in the world and what their future will be like. If you watch closely, you can see and hear where people stack the deck in their favor or interfere in their own progress.

What I have noticed, is that the things/phrases people frequently say and their behaviors which are based on their attitudes, not only reflect what is going on both from a psychological and emotional standpoint, but also the phrases themselves circle back and either limit or release a person to go onto to bigger and better life experiences.

Over the decades of personal training, I've noticed patterns in the people who seem to take to exercise and nutrition easily (regardless of their previous experiences or lack thereof) and the ones who seem to have difficulty in even comprehending what is expected of them (even if they have had numerous experiences with personal trainers).

In these next two chapters are some [generalities] which stand out for both people who lean toward positive emotional states and negative emotional states that are related to successes and failures in their chosen goals.

Again, I want to reiterate that no one is positive all the time or in all contexts (everyone experiences disappointment)...its more about a person's general nature, constitution and predisposition (whatever tendency people lean toward, when faced with challenge or disappointment), which determines how things progress and turn out after a perceived setback.

In relation to fat-loss specifically, simply staying in the game, continuing to stay in motion, instead of concluding you, *"...can't do it"* when you have feelings is the single greatest behavior that determines progress. Regardless of what you feel, simply keep going. [People who have suppressed emotions, or emotional confusion tend to conclude that since they are having feelings, they can't move forward. In attempt to control their feelings, they stop moving instead of moving and letting the feelings go, which affirms emotional paralysis].

As usual, nature always surprises and you can have a mostly positive person who has difficulty and a seeming negative person who seems to take to their workouts, with ease. A person might be positive in one area of their life but haven't cross-contextualized their positivity into other areas and that's ok, too.

The single greatest influential factor of all seems to be whether a person projects successful attainment of their goals (combination of visualizing success as already happened, combined with cultivating the emotions of achievement & faith) or projects that they're going to have a difficult time and suffer during the process.

From a personal training standpoint, negative people tend to suck energy off others around them (nature abhors a vacuum) through a misunderstanding of use of energy, while positive people tend to gain energy by giving positive energy to those around them, thereby creating space for channeling more positive energy through themselves to give to others again, in a continuous cycle. Negative people tend to use (hold energy and emotions) while positive people tend to give (release energy & emotions and move on).

Negative people tend to require more energy on the trainer's part, since negativity isn't self-sustaining...it requires others to sustain it from the outside, since the main metaphor of negativity is a lack of faith and gratitude (not necessarily in a religious manner) and ultimately, a underlying hunger for positivity in the body and mind. But, unless the change occurs from within the person, no amount of external input of positivity solves the problem, which is the result of internal choices, depending which attitudes are allowed to be at home in the mind and body. Although people will say things like, *I am what I am*, ultimately, it's a personal choice about quality of life. Some people are so addicted to negativity that they have a difficult time seeing outside the negativity itself (they identify with it and think of it as being practical).

Usually, until a person really gets that their attitude is preventing them from having the quality of life, career, health or relationships they aren't likely to change. Sometimes, people are so caught up in their ego that the more they are told that the problem is "their attitude", the more they dig their heels in and do more of the thing that is preventing them from getting what they want. Sometimes people use the results of their negative attitude to rationalize their negative attitude...in other words, they say they have to have a negative attitude because what life and others have done to them, not realizing that their attitude is attracting the people and situations that feed off negativity. I have seen people have the *"aha"* moment in this regard and turn it around.

Sometimes people simply don't know that they get to choose their attitude and their attitude affect what opportunities they have in life...when they realize they get to choose, they seemingly instantly do a 360° and their life improves dramatically over the following months and years.

Sometimes people think choosing their attitude isn't an authentic version of themselves (their identity is attached), not realizing that somewhere along the way they chose their attitude, but it became an unconscious habit they don't remember choosing, even if it began as modeling or copying their family members.

Sometimes, a person's attitude is what it is because the person concluded something about life before they had all the facts. If we conclude before we have all the facts (even though we think we have all the facts) we're essentially experiencing a misunderstanding, but perceiving we're fully informed.

Tendencies of positive-based personalities:

■ Feeling inspired and relaxed.

■ Looking forward to a bright future.

■ Anticipating and expecting success.

■ Follow directions/coachable.

■ Learn as you go and teach others.

■ Build a healthy circle of influence.

■ Finds a way. Makes the way to get it done.

■ Acknowledges feelings, but sets feelings aside and lets them go to get the workout done and put the B.N.B.B. in.

■ Surrenders to the process of the science of fat-loss. Has faith it works.

- Behaving as a victor.

- Attached to the idea of becoming happy & joyous even if they haven't figured it out.

- Identifies with success.

- Looking forward to future success.

- Names behaviors without making excuses or rationalizing.

- Feels, acknowledges, releases, *feels* lighter.

- Takes care of self, *first.*

- Consistent.

- Participates.

- Learns the differences between quality, efficiency & effectiveness versus quantity, ineffectiveness, randomness.

- Directness.

- Agreeable.

- Reasonable: Get along well with others.

- Happiness.

- Follow through.

- *"I lost another 5% last night."*

- Simply follows through.

- *"Show me what to do."*

- *"I don't really understand yet, but I take my B.N.B.B.s and exercise anyway."*

- Does the basics consistently.

- Wants to know where they aren't quite dialed in, yet.

- Proactive self care.

- *"Thank you for showing me!"*

■ Curiosity.

■ Acts on professional suggestions.

■ *"The cup is half full."*

■ Takes B.N.B.B.s daily.

■ No failure, just feedback and correction.

■ *"Every little bit adds up."*

■ Focused on fundamentals/isn't distracted.

■ Entertains the idea of tranquility, serenity, poise, composure, enthusiasm and cheerfulness.

■ Moderation in behavior.

■ Sticks to basics.

■ Forthright.

■ Optimism.

■ Spends time reminiscing about how bright their future is when they have reached their goals.

■ Behaves as if success is inevitable (develops precedence of emotional control).

■ Self-empowering behaviors.

■ *"I just do it. "*

■ Notices, acknowledges and addresses addictive behavior.

■ Goes on to master the fundamentals.

■ Consistently consume enough B.N.B.B.s the cravings stay away.

■ Notices and masters impulse control.

■ Completes and gets a new workout plan every 6-7 weeks.

■ Measures, tracks and recalculates target heart rate, body composition and calories the first of every month.

■ Attitude of re-inventing self.

Chapter conclusion:

By periodically perusing this list, you can measure the effectiveness of how well you are progressing at experiencing your emotions and letting them go versus being controlled by your emotions.

"Sov knows how to relate to his clients and get them motivated to attain their goals. Sov is outstanding at relating the individual's personal goals to the training routine. Having never been to a gym before last September ('06), Sov took an intimidating experience and turned it into something I enjoy. Sovereign cares about his clients...I have watched the other trainers work with their clients and Sovereign's interaction with his clients is 100%...I have watched other trainers be distracted with cell phones, "cruise" other gym members, etc., but Sov always gives me 100% of my time and his concentration. I AM extremely SATISFIED with the time I spend w/Sovereign & would recommend him to others..." B.D., Billings, MT

Chapter Sixteen

Qualities of Being
Emotionally Disassociated/Not Present

I want to emphasize that there isn't anything inherently wrong when we don't know how to access positive emotional states. It happens to all of us! The point being to increase your awareness of yourself, acknowledge when something is off, notice the pattern or strategy which isn't working and then through careful and consistent introspection develop emotional strategies which enable the achievements of your goals...regardless of the context. With that in mind, below is a list of some of the common negative attitudes and phrases which can interfere with progressive fat-loss progress.

■ Anxious; worry about the future (lack of presence/lack of faith).

■ Scared/fearful of change (lack of self confidence/lack of faith).

■ Doubtful/skeptical to where it interferes in simply exercising and taking the B.N.B.B.s. (arrogance)

■ Indifference (lack of presence/*dis*-associated).

■ Can't/won't take direction or stick to tasks (hasn't decided to change).

■ Takes pride in telling trainer how they didn't exercise impulse control (identity level).

■ Doesn't/won't intend to retain information that (refuting accountability).

■ Won't expand circle of influence (self-image).

■ Attached to own unhappiness (identity).

■ *"I can't..."* (self-confidence, competence, self-image).

■ Focuses on feeling feelings so much, is paralyzed...feels like they can't move forward (containin the emotions).

■ Resists simply doing exercise and nutrition (too much attention on feelings).

■ Behaves/sees self as a victim (gaining attention and energy though sympathy rather than brainstorming solutions).

■ *"Oh, whoa-is-me."* (self-pity/martyr).

■ Identifies with past failures or disappointments, think they can't surpass past or concludes that past shortcomings mean they shouldn't regroup and make another attempt, this time with professional guidance (self-image).

■ Feels, but suppresses, holds onto emotions and eats to cover up/distract from feelings (holding onto emotions rather than letting them pass and moving on).

■ Doesn't know feelings are normal, but holding them is not (need to learn to experience, keep the lesson and let go of the emotions).

■ *"I just look at food and goes to my hips!"* (lack of honesty with self).

■ Apathy (lack of presence).

■ *"I smell a cake and it sticks to my butt!"* (lack of honesty with self).

■ Insisting on a need to understand every detail before beginning...but you can't understand the thing until you complete the thing, so you don't begin (procrastination & distraction; lack of faith).

■ *"I'm doing everything right and I'm still not losing weight,"* (lack of honesty with self).

■ Keeps plans a secret; disappointed when others don't respect boundaries that you didn't speak out loud (martyr).

■ *"I don't know"* is the common response (*dis*-empowers self; instead of taking a breath, asking a question and then being patient and present and allowing the answer to come to you). If you don't know, then you aren't responsible for the truth. *The truth will set you free.*

■ Attempts to take care of others' feelings, but ignores self-care (lack of self-worth/co-dependency).

■ Inconsistent effort (lack of decision to succeed).

■ Lacks participation (wants Fat-loss to be done to them or for them) [side-effect belief as a result of taking too much care of others/co-dependency].

■ Exhibits half-effort, values quantity over quality, does random exercises rather than specific strategies and counts random activity as effort without results, then subsequently complains that nothing works (lack of commitment/lack of B.N.B.B.s).

■ Indirect communications (lack of accountability & disrespect of self).

■ *"I was just going to have a little taste and then I ate the whole thing!"* (malnourished).

■ Generally disagreeable (lack of commitment & focus).

■ Wants the magic pill (lack of honesty with self).

■ Lacks follow through (lack of decision to change).

■ *"I didn't lose any weight today...I don't think it works, can't we do something different?"* (attempting to get permission to not adhere to the program; lack of commitment).

■ Victim mentality: Over identifies with what happened in the past/ doesn't make room for or allow the future.

■ Argumentative (malnourished, lack of focus, lack of decision to change)

■ Won't stick to a basic plan consistently (lack of commitment).

■ Doesn't want constructive criticism/doesn't want to be accountable/not interested or invested (not coachable/un-committed).

■ Avoids self-care (self-worth).

■ *"Don't tell me what to do!"* (accountability; misunderstands responsibility to self).

■ *Dis*-interested. (lack of commitment).

■ Excuses why they couldn't do the thing (lack of follow through).

■ *"The cup is half empty,"* (bad attitude).

■ *"How come I can't eat just one?"* (malnourished/lack of B.N.B.B.s).

■ Allowing past experiences to define/limit you in the future (self-image; stuck in the past/lack of goals).

■ Can't remember to take B.N.B.B.s (malnourished/B.N.B.B.s).

■ Beats up on self-degrading self-talk (self-image/self-esteem).

■ *"I'm not getting results fast enough,"* (misunderstands commitment & follow through; hasn't applied self to long-term goals before; wants a quick fix for a lifestyle problem).

■ Won't stick to fundamentals, easily distracted (lack of commitment).

■ Lack of moderation in behavior (all or nothing). (compulsion/impulsive/malnourished).

■ *"Do I have to?"* (lack of self-worth).

■ So afraid of the idea of addiction that won't acknowledge if addiction is a factor in their own life. Improvement is difficult if addictive behaviors aren't addressed, even if the addiction is sugar (denial/avoidance/addiction).

■ Lack of consistency with fundamentals prevents progressing to advanced techniques (inconsistent).

■ Skips workouts and subsequently doesn't follow through to update workout plan every 6-7 weeks (accountability).

■ Attitude of wanting to stay the same but get different results (selfishness/unwilling to earn it/entitlement/arrogance).

■ *"I'm an exception to the rules...I'm so different that exercise and nutrition don't apply to me."* (denial).

■ *"...a glass of wine!...I drink a bottle every night."* (addiction and malnutrition).

■ *"What's the use?"* (learned helplessness/lack of follow-through).

■ *"Yay, yay...I know all that but tell me what works,"* (believes in short cuts/denial).

■ *"You told me to ride the bike for 20 minutes...I rode it for 60 minutes,"* (Hurry up/procrastinate/self-sabotage/un-coachable).

■ *"You can't make me eat,"* (wants attention/immaturity).

■ *"You can't make me take care of myself,"* (self-loathing/polar responder/boomerang/co-dependency).

■ Feels, suppresses and holds inside/acts out self-sabotage/hurts self directly or passively through neglect (lack of personal accountability/inner-conflict).

■ Focused on immediate gratification versus long-term satisfaction & fulfillment (compulsive/impulsive/immaturity/entitlement).

■ Rationalizes poor behaviors/rationalizes procrastination (makes excuses/lack of accountability to self).

■ Prioritizes feeling for others. Tries to prevent others having feelings, e.g. sadness, disappointment, etc., (co-dependent/martyr).

■ Inconsistency (lack of habit).

■ *"Wait, stop...not so fast...too fast,"* (traumatized/shell-shocked/lack of integration of past/sorting/debriefing).

■ *"I don't know what to do,"* (malnourished/lack of personal responsibility/B.N.B.B.s).

■ Avoidance of accountability.

■ Disagreeable (malnourished).

■ Unreasonable: Demands a lot of others, but doesn't hold self-accountable.

■ Manipulates situation to create distance from others (fear of intimacy).

■ Depressed (recycling and/or inordinate amount of focus on the past experiences) or what could have been or should have been.

■ Anxiety (reminiscing about the future/imagining what might happen).

■ Flakey, fickle, non-complaint (lack of responsibility/immaturity).

■ Exaggeration of affects of moderate food intake after excessive consumption" -says they had a little and gained weight but really had a lot and gained weight from excess (dishonesty).

■ Not naming malnutrition-based cravings, *"Last night I was dying for some ice cream,"* (malnutrition/B.N.B.B.s/boomerang).

■ *"I paid $5,000 for personal training...when does the fat go away?"* (entitlement combined with lack of intention/unreasonable expectations)

■ *"Help me...no, no, not like that,"* (control issues).

■ Dishonest or lack of accountability: *"I don't know why I did that,"* (take a breath, get present, pay attention to yourself, and figure it out so you have it for the future).

■ *"I want to lose weight, but I don't want to exercise or take supplements...tell me what to do,"* (unreasonable expectations).

■ *"I'm too busy,"* (lack of priorities).

■ Pessimism (malnutrition).

■ Shame & remorse (habitual triggers for compulsive consumption without conscious interruption).

■ *"You can't make me eat,"* (inner-conflict/trying to get attention for negative behaviors/attempting independence but *mis*-understanding what independence means: responsibility to take care of self-accompanies independence).

■ *"I don't like people I'm paying to help me telling me what to do!"* (immaturity/attention seeking/striving for inappropriate boundaries).

■ Does the opposite of the what the professionals they have asked for help and guidance suggest. (opposite response/polar/boomerang)

■ *"I can't remember,"* (emotional fogginess/lack of commitment/malnutrition/B.N.B.B.s).

■ *"I was just going buy a cake for a friend but then I ate the whole thing,"* (dishonesty/malnutrition/B.N.B.B.s).

■ *"How come I can't eat just one,"* (cravings/lack of B.N.B.B.s in brain).

■ Attitude of being the one and only exception to the laws of nature. ...*"the rules don't apply to me,"* (arrogance = fear + anger & resentment).

■ *"A glass of wine?...I drink a bottle every night...isn't a little wine okay?"* (addiction & denial).

■ All or nothing behavior (lack of moderation & self-defeatist attitude).

■ *"Yay, yay...I know all that but tell me what works,"* (information-junkie to facilitate procrastination).

■ *"What's the use?"* (learned helplessness).

■ Beats-up-on-self to rationalize nutritional cheating and inactivity (addicted to negativity & self-loathing).

■ *"I don't want to get to muscular."* and or *"I don't want to cut back food, I'll become anorexic,"* (irrational excuses as procrastination & distraction to avoid fundamentals).

■ *"Is now the time I can have some S.A.D.C.R.A.P.?"* (self-loathing).

■ Perceives the fitness-lifestyle as their happiness being taken away from them versus creating and brining in a bright future.

■ *"Too much is never enough,"* (masochism/self-punishment/self-loathing).

■ Says dietary supplements are extreme, but can't figure out why they aren't burning fat (denial).

■ "The *Hurry UP!* and Procrastinate" phenomena among fat-loss clients (self-sabotage).

(Since compulsion & impulsiveness are two common traits of clients who haven't been able to stick with a program, [to allow a program to work for them], one of the common traits is they want priority care, push the trainer to hurry and get their program set up and once they have it they begin picking the program apart. Unbelievably, and to my astonishment, one of the most common traits among people who want the "secret pill" to fat-loss is they truly believe they are going to find someone who will teach them how to keep doing the lifestyle they've been doing that got them fat, but get all the benefits of someone applying a fitness-lifestyle.

These are the people who insist you're ruining their lives by taking away the ingredients they rely on in their addiction and the S.A.D.C.R.A.P.

One of the surest markers of someone who isn't going to follow through is the client who waits until they are clinically obese, then insists they want you to train them, but as soon as you make them a priority they begin making up reasons why they can't do this, can't do that and insist you have to remove the parts of the training that applies to them and their habits. They essentially want all the parts that make it a fat-loss program removed. Once you insist they have to learn the fundamentals and the program was designed with their particulars in mind, they begin attempting to attack the professional credibility of the trainer.

In these cases, I bless them and send them on their way. Until they are willing to learn the fundamentals of a fitness-lifestyle, no one can help them. These are the same people who have a long list of trainers and health care providers who didn't have what it took to help them.

■ Dismisses guidance from trainer. *"My trainer told me to take the B.N.B.B.s but I don't believe him/her...I just don't think it's that important."*

■ Doesn't schedule appointment with self to update body composition, resting heart rate (target heart rate) nor calorie requirements, then complains their results are inconsistent, nor get professional help to do so (lack of commitment & accountability).

At some point, in order to achieve goals, we have to exercise emotional integrity and override what we feel like doing in the moment to get the big pay-off we want in the long-run. In some ways, this can be thought of as an emotional-awakening.

When you begin a well-designed exercise and nutrition program, it's not likely to feel natural, since its different than what you've been doing. This is one place where it will take a few weeks for your new program to feel natural and one place where you'll want to simply stick to the plan and follow through, while noticing and acknowledging but setting your feelings aside, since they'll likely try to convince you to attend to them, rather than your program. That means you'll want to get used to what you're doing feeling unnatural at first and proceeding on faith.

It's common when a person who pays an unhealthy level of attention to how they feel in every minute (and subsequently attempt to avoid those feelings) and then proceed to find a new, better trainer, they are excited until the trainer guides and suggests behaviors which will short-circuit the self-defeating behavior(s). In other words, in an effort to perfect-the-neurosis, they force the trainer (for holding them accountable) to behaviors that will help the client get what they hired the trainer, doctor, coach, etc. I've even had a client discontinue training when I insist the take the time to stretch (avoiding getting present in their body).

This type of behavior occurs with clients/patients in every profession and is often referred to as the patient being non-compliant (relates to the patient or client being in what's referred to as the [pre-contemplation phase] (of behavioral change). *More on this in the six stages of behavioral change.* Until one is fully committed, they refuse to do the behaviors to get what they say they want...as long as people still believe they can get what they want without doing the actions required, they remain in a state where they think they can out-negotiate the laws of nature and simultaneously blame others or make excuses why they haven't gotten the results they want.

Chapter conclusion:

By periodically perusing this list, you can measure the effectiveness of how well you are progressing at experiencing your emotions and letting them go versus being controlled by your emotions.

Well, it's almost been two weeks since I started following your recommendations on diet and exercise. I'm feeling really good! The hardest part is easing up on my riding intensity. I used to ride 20 miles in about an hour (ave heart rate was around 160 or higher). Now when I ride I keep it at or under 146 and I can't believe how much better I feel. I don't feel worn out when I'm done and feel like I could ride for hours at that pace. My morning rides last about an hour and cover about 14 miles. I've also been on the resistance plan 3X a week and feeling stronger already. I started adding 20 min of cardio this past week after

Chapter Seventeen

The Six Stages Of Behavioral Change

When we take a good look at the differences between the people who decide on a goal, follow through and reach their goals versus people who have goals but can't seem to follow through, we can compare a person's behaviors with what stage of behavioral change they are in, at the moment. By determining what stage of change a person is in, at the moment helps us to know what kind of work needs to happen to help you go to the next stage. In other words, if you really haven't decided to move forward then it doesn't make sense to tell you what it takes to succeed...you haven't decided to succeed yet!

Knowing what stage a person is at requires asking questions also known as an interview or initial consultation.

I don't know what these stages were originally outlined for, but it seems every kind of health care provider eventually learns about them, often when they are talking to a colleague or mentor, when they are trying to figure out what might be missing within a client or patient's progress.

What that means is that most coaches, trainers, doctors, physician assistants, physical therapists, etc., get tons of education, looking forward to helping people in need. Unfortunately, there's a significant portion of the population who will complain about their situation, but when it comes to doing the things that are proven to help, they disappear. This can leave professionals scratching their head since they are doing everything in their power to help people and it's during this time that health care providers learn that it doesn't matter how much professional training they have. If a person hasn't decided to change and then back it up with consistent action there's nothing else you can do for them. You can't make a person change. You can't make a person improve something they won't acknowledge their responsibility in. You can't make a person heal, who is emotionally stuck...it's an inside job. If you've ever visited a health care provider and they seem short-tempered, impatient and as if your story isn't that important it could very well mean they've had more than their share of patients who complain about their situation, want to go on and on about how much they are suffering, but then won't do a simple step that's suggested. Often these kinds of patients come back again and again, with the same complaints, but not taking responsibility for the situation. An alternate behavior would be to simply do the thing the health professional suggests and if you want to do research for alternate modalities do so, but to do nothing but keep complaining is a definition of insanity (doing the same thing over and over but expecting a different result).

One of the coping mechanisms trainers and health care providers eventually come across is the model of The Stages of Behavioral Change (The Transtheretical Model). This model helps because it describes the behaviors that match the current mind set where a person is. In other words, the client's behavior is a better indicator than what the client insists or says their goals are. If the goals and the stage of behavioral change are not in alignment, then they will often sign up, join or get associated gear, but not follow through. This model helps you know if the weakness is a lack of education, training or caring on the professional's part or if the problem is with the client/patient's commitment level and ability to follow through on what they say they want. There are a lot of cases where people's brains are functioning so low, from chronic malnutrition, that they can't take in the very information that would help them the most...cognitive-function (ability to reason) and will-power are [functions] of the consistently, well-nourished brain. If you don't nourish yourself there's nothing else anyone can do for you...*no amount of prescription drugs will make up for a problem that is based in lack of nutrition and exercise*...a significant emotional stumbling block for many because they don't want to hear that...the brain that wants sugar, doesn't want to hear about nutrition density. You can't outrun poor nutrition with any amount of exercise, since nutrition is required to utilize fat for energy and to get the body-fat level to 20% or less.

Keep in mind that people who have the most trouble reaching goals often don't realize that reaching their goals involves not just thinking or talking about the goal, but backing up the goal with very specific actions (which they might not know what those actions are) or even actions that they have to learn in order to reach their goals. "Wanting" the goal isn't enough to attain it. When I began college, I had to learn how to learn since really hadn't had much experience at applying myself academically...I had to change and improve as a person, just to engage in the process of learning in order to reach my goal as a helicopter pilot. I was the first in my family to attend college, so I had never seen anyone studying the way I needed to successfully participate in college.

Part of the common problem is that we see and hear successful people on TV and media once they have already succeeded and a lot of the public doesn't know the extra-ordinary amount of energy and sacrifice that has gone into the accomplishment and they think reaching a goal comes from simply saying you have the goal and wanting it.

The six stages:

Pre-contemplation is the where the person hasn't considered needing to change their behaviors, didn't know that reaching a goal would require behaving differently or didn't know that to get different results you have to behave differently than the behaviors that got you where you are. Sometimes people around us might make comments that we need to "change" but in this stage, there's an aspect of it being just outside awareness or we think we can keep going how we are and everything will be fine, or we'll reach the goal doing what hasn't worked before. In this stage, people will say they want to lose weight, set surface goals but then resist and resent and feedback or guidance that would actually facilitate them reaching the goals. It's not uncommon for people to think that by paying a personal trainer, the trainer is going to do something "to them" that will make the fat go away like a salon treatment or something.

An aspect of this stage is that familiarity with what the person knows and is comfortable with takes precedence over doing new behaviors. In this stage, the person believes they can keep doing fat building behaviors but somehow, magically burn fat. There's an aspect of denial, through naivety in this stage.

Clients in the pre-contemplation stage will have a look of surprise or disgust when the personal trainer they approached for help starts discussing the frequency of the exercise program or nutritional habits required to reach the goals they insist they want and re ready for!

Contemplation stage is where the person hast started to realize that if they really want to attain the goal, they might have to do things differently...maybe. For the trainer and health care providers, it's important to note that in this stage there's no guarantees...just because the client or provider knows "about" this stage or recognizes it, doesn't mean the client/patient will suddenly change and do what's expected of them. The time it takes from contemplation to determination is indefinable...meaning the client might be in this stage for a moment or the rest of their life (NLP, hypnosis & motivational interviewing are three great tools to help clients/patients get past this stage). The more competent the professional help they seek, the easier it will likely be to transition from one stage to the next.

One thing that speeds the process at this stage is when someone becomes conscious of the behavior needed is outside them (*"...some people take dietary supplements."*) to a thing they embody and identify with (*"...dietary supplements make burning fat easier for me."*). Although there are common denominator qualities among people who go from pre-contemplation, to contemplation and onto determination, there are cases where "the straw that breaks the camel's back" is something simple and unexpected, yet holds great meaning to the person. In other words, when they say what it was that caused change or changed within them, to the listener it doesn't sound significant enough, yet from a tonality there is obvious significance and leaves the trainer or practitioner thinking, *"Huh, how come I didn't think of that?"* Often, I refer to this as "encoded-emotionality" since, from the outside, it doesn't add up, like *"I stuck to my exercise program because 1+1=7."*

The phrase "it doesn't add up", but somehow they attach meaning to a nonsensical statement and it facilitates progress and that is good enough as long as the statement reflects something they have control over. If the reason is based on something outside their control, or other people then if the situation changes they have lost the thing that was making it possible to maintain behavioral engagement.

One of the potentially confusing things about fat-loss is that the science works (exercise and nutrition), but the emotional aspect has to be justified by each person to their own satisfaction. Trainers and health care providers can help people sort out their own reasons in the contemplation stages, but can't be attached to "how" it plays out...it doesn't matter how it happens as long as the client does their exercise and nutrition.

If the trainer and client are simply demonstrating leader and follower roles, progress is sure. But when the client hasn't done the work to really be ready to engage they often try to get the trainer to follow them, to the place we already know doesn't achive mutual outcomes.

Often, people think by buying a personal trainer or a gym membership they'll feel different about going to the gym, but it doesn't do anything since the change hasn't happened on the inside, yet. The fitness-lifestyle interferes with the fat-lifestyle and that often comes as a surprise to new clients. This eludes to the concept of "criteria". In other words, the thing that holds enough importance to cause internal change in motivation that leads to new behavior(s). Sometimes the critical criteria surfaces spontaneously from within and sometimes it comes through motivational interviewing (hint) by the trainer and health care providers.

In my experience, I would guess about 60% of people who join a gym or seek personal training have made the internal adjustments to simply begin doing the thing and about 40% need more help working through pre-contemplation and contemplation stages to get where they'll be ready to begin. Statistically, for people who join a gym in January, about 60% have quit within three months, due to lack of results. I believe because they think they can do random activity and get the results they want, skip the nutrition and forego getting professional training thinking they know better.

Within three months, a fully committed person who is doing the three parts of nutrition as I suggest, could burn 36 to 60 pounds of fat.

Gym members watch other members doing activities and tell themselves the people are just, *"...doing stuff"* and conclude just doing stuff or being "around" the equipment produces the results they want. It takes about three months for people to realize random activity doesn't work, but then they're so burned out from not getting results that they talk themselves out of getting professional help, not realizing they will take that training with them for the rest of their lives...*how do you put a price on that?*

Once a person has worked through the process of finding/making conscious their own motivation and connecting with it the process can be repeated and in other contexts/goals. This is part of what is referred to is self-empowerment and cross-contextualiztion.

Clients in the contemplation stage will begin to participate and show up for workouts, but may bounce back and forth from pre-contemplation to contemplation as they are working to convince themselves to give up the fat-lifestyle in exchange for the fitness-lifestyle. When they aren't completely convinced that they will feel better, look better and reach their goals it's not likely they will allocate time, energy and resources to something they don't have faith in. Whether they do or not get results depends on how well their exercise and nutrition program is designed. I personally like people to begin seeing and feeling results within the first three days of beginning. If the client hasn't burned at least 12 pounds of fat within the first month, something is off, either in the design, the demonstration or the execution of the program.

I've actually heard trainers say they don't want their clients to get results too quickly, for fear of the client discontinuing training thinking they can do it on their own. I've also seen trainers who don't know what they're doing say that result within three months isn't reasonable.

If the exercise and nutrition program are properly designed, 12 to 20 pounds of fat-loss per month is reasonable, sustainable and health building.

Determination stage is when the person starts getting prepared mentally and emotionally for doing the actions which will hopefully get them their goal(s). This is the place where inertia (lack of activity) has to be overcome...the place where you have to force yourself to start, even though it might be unfamiliar and uncomfortable. With people who have tried to burn fat and get healthy before and didn't follow through for whatever reason, they don't really exhibit determination until they start getting results they consider significant. In other words, they might show up, require some pushing, but once they begin seeing and feeling results, it's as though a fire has been ignited and they realize their effort is causing change/improvements (if the exercise and nutrition programs were designed and carried out properly).

Once you've made the decision to begin, the quantity of drive to get the thing done is only limited by 1) How well you connect to what you want 2) How much you prioritize resources for it in your life (time, energy & money) 3) How efficiently you connect positive emotions of accomplishment, with envisioning the goal having already been attained (future-pacing) and 4) How well you execute doing what you've been taught without skipping, subsituting or altering anything.

People who see the goal as accomplished as they begin and combine it with the positive emotions of having completed the thing (as though it already occurred) show a seeming endless supply of physical, mental and emotional energy to get the thing done.

For people who study this kind of phenomena (future-pacing), it appears as though the amount of energy a person has for a goal is determined and distributed [by the future] not by [the present time] where the person is today, as we most commonly perceive. Instead of viewing it as a question of how much you'll *have to do*, you'll be more likely to succeed at anything (and find great ease in the process) by envisioning what you want to be, have or experience, and connecting emotions to the finished thing as though its already accomplished. By doing so you just have to jump through the hoops known as required activities to make room for the thing to come to pass.

The more you create the feelings of gratitude and faith "as if" or assume the thing has happened the less actual energy and exertion you'll perceive needing to spend. It's not a thing you have to talk about, because being grateful is strictly a doing thing...an action...a behavior...an internal state that affects the outside world. I think this is one of the dearest held phenomena of time, and a reason why life seems to come easier for some people.

Action stage means behavior. Behavior is doing. Doing *consistently* is what gets the results you insist you want. Repeating what works. A common misconception for people who have had an ongoing challenge to burn fat, let alone maintain it, is the realization that *it's all about you!* Your success or lack thereof is entirely based on you following through on the action that is specifically designed to burn fat...not random activity you think others are doing or what you would rather be doing to distract yourself.

People can bounce back and forth or regress between stages as behavioral change isn't necessarily a straight line of progress. Part of what can occur is when someone has an unconscious belief (e.g. *"I'll always be fat,"* or *"I failed before, so I'll fail again."*). Part of this phenomena is because as the client experiences progress that conflicts with what they believed was possible, the ideas/beliefs surface to tell the person that they can't do it or that they can't make it. This is a place where successful people simply show up for their workouts and continue with their nutrition regardless of what they mind is telling them to the contrary, e.g. set the emotions aside and do the work anyway (feel the fear and do it anyway).

The successful person notices and challenges what negative messages their mind is giving, but continues with action (they separate thoughts from feelings: clarity)...it's in the consistent small actions that add up to cumulative benefits where life transforms and you see what you're truly capable of.

One way to know what your unconscious beliefs about your success are is to make positive, affirmative statements to yourself, e.g. *"I have burned 20 pounds of fat this month,"* and then listen to what self-talk comes up. If there's anything but positive, it indicates where you want to focus your energy to root out the beliefs that are counterproductive to your goals, yet interfere with your behavior at an unconscious level.

The unsuccessful person listens to the negative messages but instead of challenging them, takes action/does behaviors that match the negative messages (collapsing thoughts and emotions; confusion), resulting in simple neglect of the exercise and nutrition programs.

More often than not, people who haven't been able to burn fat correctly or consistently either believe/think that something is going to be done "to them" or believe that by simply being around a trainer or "around" exercise equipment they'll burn fat! Nothing is further from the truth. If you're not sure, do a web search for some of the first couple episodes from each of the 16 seasons of *The Biggest Loser* TV show. Usually in the first couple episodes of each season you see people who have nowhere else to turn, are in grave danger since they are so obese but want to give up during the first workouts. And they're surprised that they have to do the work, even though they knew about the show by watching the show *("I'm an exception to the rules.")*.

A commonality with people who have struggled to get rid the fat is a disconnect related to connecting with the part of themselves that makes things happen. Will-power? *Maybe*, but will-power seems to be a function of the brain which is nourished properly. You'll hear and recognize malnourished people say they don't have any will-power! So, people who haven't used their personal power to apply physical exertion to make a thing happen, they are often very surprised that the fat-loss isn't going to be done *"to them"*... that they have to exert themselves to change direction from gaining fat to using fat for energy. They don't know that burning fat, getting lean and becoming healthier requires specific, strategic, consistent action. In my approach, that means three, 50-minute sessions of resistance-training per week, three 20, minute sessions of fat-burning aerobic training per week and complete nutrition 1) Whole-foods 2) Functional-foods and 3) Certain dietary supplements at certain times (B.N.B.B.s).

The reason these principles are repeated so much throughout the book is that the people who need this information the most tend to glean over, rationalize or dismiss the key points in hope that no one will notice they are skipping the keys that make the difference. Through repetition, it's easier to accept ideas that conflict with beliefs about what a person will achieve.

It's not uncommon for people to say, *"I just want to get started, but I don't want to do resistance training, cardio or the nutrition stuff...just the other stuff."*...What other stuff?

Maintenance stage is where you have reached the fat-loss goals you wanted from the beginning (20% or less) and you have moved into maintaining that level of success as well as refining your practice to "dial-it-in". In this stage you keep getting the same or better results with less energy than it took to get there (greater efficiency). For a lot of people, once they achieve their primary goal, they start thinking about doing events like 5k & 10k walk and runs or other kinds of fitness/athletic events. In these cases, you'll need to get your body-fat lower to do well and perform at your best. Simply keep doing what you've been doing to get your body composition to the 10%-15% range.

A key point in progress is when a person begins to see themselves (self-image) as athletic or as an athlete or even fit. If you can see yourself as athletic or at least a fitness buff, your workouts will become easier as your self-image is matching your investments of time, energy and money.

The main misconception that interferes with the maintenance stage is that once you reach [preliminary] goals you "get to" go back to the lifestyle that got you fat in the first place as if some kind of reward. OR, as soon as you begin to get some results, you forget about the goals you initially set and begin idling. Being lean and healthy is a lifestyle the same as getting fat was a lifestyle. People who don't understand the lifestyle concept think in terms of rewarding themselves for doing what they should have been living anyway. The more undernourished a person, the more they think this way since the undernourished mind craves the payoff of junk food. Undernourished people aren't able to think and process that the payoff is the journey itself nor that getting rid all that fat IS the payoff, since the brain is still preoccupied with the attempting to get nourished through junk food. The undernourished brain is lacking the key nutrition it needs and is waiting for the quick-fix which shows up as behaviorally as though healthy/good behavior is supposed to be *rewarded* (it's not) with unhealthy S.A.D.C.R.A.P. (this is really malformed thinking). How this shows up is when people who begin with body-fat greater than 20% and they notice their clothes begin to "feel" more loose and they stop following through, having lost sight of their goals and the importance of consistency.

I had one client who was in the 36% body composition fat range. As soon as she got signed up for training, her first questions were about when she gets to start having cheat days with her nutrition. At 36% body-fat, the person has so much fat they are essentially a walking time bomb. To be in that much disrepair and be concerned about when you're going to get to start eating S.A.D.C.R.A.P. again indicates addictive type habits.

The most effective way I have observed successful people prepare for these six stages is to assure they have enough B.N.B.B.s on board, regardless of how much a beginner can rationalize nutrition that they are convinced they don't need! A beginner being anyone who hasn't reached their goals and maintained them for the rest of their life. If they haven't maintained it successfully, it simply means they have taken a run at it before, but were missing one or more components which permit sustainability.

Nutritional density isn't a "rational" process, since the brain that is undernourished won't say, *"Get the B.N.B.B.s"*, it will simply show you by what your hands grab and put in your mouth and by what consumables you bring into your house...*S.A.D.C.R.A.P.* Even for people who get the B.N.B.B.s and get amazing results, if they don't work through the inner-conflicts of their self-image, they'll often start and stop...when the ego isn't getting its way, the person will find it difficult to be consistent even though the actions match what they insist are their goals. And that's where forcing yourself to do correct actions until they become a habit and feel familiar come into play...*that's what successful people do!* They force themselves to do the actions to get their outcomes and are grateful they know what to do.

The more consistent you are at putting the B.N.B.B.s in your body every day, whether you think you want to or not, the easier and more effortless maintenance mode is. It's as clear as night and day. Mood is a direct influence on sticking with your program and mood is controlled by the mount of the nutritional density you put in your body.

The better you feel the easier it is to do your program and how you "feel" is based on how nourished your brain is.

Chapter conclusion:

By identifying what stage of behavioral change you're in, you can accurately decipher what actions are next and what you have to do to move to the next stage. In other words, does the person need to do more counseling or cognitive work to clear up inner-conflict before beginning to workout? Do they need to get their blood work done to check their physical health to see for themselves the effects of their current lifestyle? Often people who really need to burn fat are in denial and until they really get in touch with the seriousness of the situation, they tell themselves they don't really need to lose weight…they think fat-loss is optional. If you're doing actions which are a mismatch for where you are on the continuum of behavioral change (difference between how you say you want to change and your internal/unconscious motivation to stay the same) then it's like the program might not makes sense...*like someone insisting you eat, when you aren't hungry.*

Often trainers and practitioners get confused because a person can be in pre-contemplation stage, but easily make an appointment or pay for a gym membership and training, which you could think is determination stage...but it isn't necessarily. In the first two stages, people will often do *determination* and *action* behaviors to find out how it "felt" and what emotions they feel as a result.

If the "feelings" they get from *determination* and *action* don't match their unconscious beliefs or self-image about themselves or what they are capable of the person may retreat, flake-out or disappear (cognitive dissonance). Hopefully, they go away and examine what they experienced, so they can work through it to move forward, but more often than not, people keep taking runs at fat-loss without knowing to address their mind and emotions. The most common result is added body-fat every time the person begins and doesn't follow through.

Moving through the stages can happen spontaneously without discussion or cognitive sorting, but if there seems to be some kind of resistance to moving forward, it could be a mismatch of where you (the client) is and what the trainer/practitioner is suggesting as the next behavior required for achievement and progress.

"Hi there Sov, thanks for sending that book along-I just finished reading it!! Tons of information there, I love it too, want to keep learning everything, so I can really be my best self. Gotta' tell you, last night I think I spent my whole night dreaming of this program!! and it has been on my mind quite a bit all day. I can definitely see a difference in my balance and strength, and I do believe my technique is improving also-better body control for exercises, more muscle strength, and more confidence in the gym, especially in the weight room. Thank you again for ALL your time and expertise that you share with me, Sov. It really does me good to talk with you, I seem to do so much better when we talk. You have such a positive energy about you, it helps to keep me focused. Just wanted to share something with you…-I saw my weight loss doctor yesterday, and I asked her about testing my blood, so I could get all my numbers for cholesterol, etc. So, they drew blood, and they just called to give me the results. I was quite pleased with everything, but here they are: Total cholesterol is 145; LDL is 76.4; HDL is 53; triglycerides are 78; and A1C level is 5.8. Blood pressure is 118/77; and still sitting at 58 pounds gone. Now let's compare these numbers to 2 years ago, when they initially did blood tests: Cholesterol was 157; LDL was 87.6; HDL was 44; triglycerides were 127; and my A1C was terrible at 6.5. Blood pressure was terrible, 140/90. So, this is real progress, what is not readily visible to people. I am very excited to see such good results, it shows that my effort is really paying off. Just goes to show that education and consistency plus dedication to change does produce results!!Thought you would like to hear this news. Thanks for helping me, I appreciate it more than you know!! Take care"

E.S., Billings, MT

Chapter Eighteen

Feeling Versus Being Rational

When the emotions aren't properly managed (live the experience and release the emotions), for whatever reason or duration, people generally feel as though they can't be themselves (living a distance from themselves). A lot of the self-improvement programs around refer to this as being your genuine/your authentic-self. Sometimes the whole suppression affect begins in an overbearing household where showing or expressing was discouraged (common in families with addiction & co-dependency). Sometimes it's when certain family members aren't comfortable with or lack coping skills in relation to emotions. Sometimes it's in relation to extreme stress or trauma that happens once or chronically over a period of time. Sometimes it's a side effect of the "elephant in the room" where a pattern of not talking about the problem spills over, to others where they lack the concept of talking about key issues, common in households with addiction. And sometimes it's just a misunderstanding with the self about your role in the world and what is permissible. Nevertheless, if someone isn't expressing and that goes on and on, they'll often subconsciously find a way to *have* their way, even if it really isn't representative of what they want...(indirect expression).

An example would be if during political elections, a person really knew candidate "A" represents them and their interests best, but instead of being direct about who they want to vote for they vote for candidate "B", whose principles actually represent the opposite of their interest...they vote for the person who is the opposite of who they want because they don't allow themselves the freedom to express...*and insist that's their candidate*. Sound familiar?

When this process of not expressing goes on for time, it's like a pressure cooker with a blocked release valve...the pressure is going to come out whether in a healthy, balanced way or not is the question. Often the emotions just come out in a weird way rather than an explicitly-destructive manner. Eventually, as a person finds ways to continue perfecting their neurosis (establish an unhealthy habit that is so complex, no one could figure it out if they wanted to: *a nervous complex that is strategically perfect in nature*...every time any professional comes close to a diagnosis, the symptoms change in nature and location...*a mystery!*) the expression that does come out isn't really a clear representation of them...*irrationality.* Sometimes clients/patients study the limitations of an emotionally-based *dis*-ease in order to make it unchangeable, so no medical provider can affect it (criteria of safe feeling in the short-term versus goal of long-term health).

Ultimately, when this process is enabled to go on and on for years, the person has relinquished so much latitude to being run by their emotions instead of having the experience and releasing the emotions, eventually the dynamics take on a life of their own and the longer it goes on, the less choice the person has...*the thinking rational-mind has been relinquished to an unsorted/unsortable complex of emotional-content that more or less just free associates off itself.* Remember that in a lot of cases, people suppress emotional-content to protect themselves from the perception of what they imagine they might experience when they stop suppressing and simply exercise and get their nutrition. Without adequate awareness, all efforts, both conscious and subconscious will be toward the outcome of suppression.

A lot of times when you hear me talk about "pet-nutritional theories", I'm also referring to people who have the irrationality-complex going on, since they are in such a suppressive habit, they exercise "choice" by choosing or doing a diet that actually [under] nourishes their brain and body even more...a form of "control" not unlike other eating disorders. They can insist they are taking care of themselves when in actuality they are deficient in iron, B vitamins and many other B.N.B.B.s as an indirect way of amplifying the suppression...effectively using nutritional science to perfect the neurosis...amplifying the "checking-out" *dis*-associative process.

With people in this state, they'll, in one minute tell you they are anemic (deficient of nutrients), that that's why they are tired and pale...and the next minute insist you should be on the same diet and that it's the diet they have their child on...*did you get that?*..it's not improving the blood chemistry, but they want others to get on it?

So, what you'll see is that people who insist on putting off their emotional health, either leaving it to chance or passive-aggressively permitting it, eventually their emotions are controlling them to the point where they can't sort experiences out or make sense of anything...*irrational.* They'll dispute science, they'll insist you're the only one that can help them, refuse to do anything that could help them *("...because it doesn't make sense to me,")* when in reality, exercise and nutrition *ONLY* make sense to the people *doing* it...discussion is often procrastination.

In these cases, you just have to pray for the person and send them on their way, if they aren't willing to get professional help. It's not likely that without getting their emotions sorted out that anyone will be able to help them and until they get real with themselves, if they aren't willing to simply do their workouts (with or without a trainer) and get the B.N.B.B.s everyday no amount of discussion will do them any service. They have effectively boxed themselves into where their emotions are so unsorted that the outside world doesn't make sense and they insist that everyone else isn't making sense. If they allowed the process to go on until hormonal changes are happening, the process is only compounded, since hormones affect thought and clarity as well. When this sort of process is allowed to go on, the people tend to believe they are an exception to the rules of nature, and that's a mirror to the fact that suppression does defy the natural laws of nature...experience and let it go...move on to the next experience. Suppression causes an internal state of being stuck in time, so anything that is communicated for the sake of help, won't make sense since it is occurring in present time, not where the suppression is in time.

An example of this phenomena in action is the classic addiction cycle where the addict denies they have an addiction, so they can't accept seeking help for the addiction. The breakdown is in the addict comprehending they have a problem, convincing themselves they are in control and consequently being unable to accept the suggestions that are possible solutions, since they deny the problem (The six stages of behavioral change). The addiction being the current complex of how they are coping with an aspect of life and the solution which takes away the coping mechanism being the thing they deny at all cost.

Whether alcohol, drugs, sugar, salt, junk food or lack of proper nutrition and exercise, the qualities and characteristics of addiction are similar and recognizable on the outside if not by the person who has the dependency.

Sort your emotions out and the outside world will make more sense.

Chapter conclusion:

Exercise and nutrition don't make sense until you stick to them long enough to see the results of sticking to them!

"Went and had a full metabolic panel done and everything came out fantastic. My doctor said, "I'm not giving you any advice, just keep doing whatever you're doing. I'm so proud and happy for you!" Since then I have tried to ignore the naysayers. I do reach out for help to make sure I'm going down the right path as this is all pretty foreign to me. And that's why I appreciate YOU! Even when your advice isn't what I want to hear, I listen because I know you know much more than I do. And I want real, lasting and healthy results! Since following your guidelines I've lost more fat, gained more muscle, brought my resting heart rate way down, stabilized my blood sugar (I was hypoglycemic to the point of passing out), regulated my blood pressure (was also regularly low 80/40), increased my energy, cut anxiety down so much that I don't even take my natural anxiety supplements anymore. Decreased cravings for unhealthy foods, but do indulge once in a while without guilt. :) I feel happier, stress doesn't get to me as badly. I'm not feeling the same negative feelings. My whole body chemistry has improved so much.
S.C, Seattle

Chapter Nineteen

A Word On Addiction To S.A.D.C.R.A.P.

S.A.D.C.R.A.P. stands for *Standard American Diet of Continuously & Repetitively Advertised Products.* Essentially, what I'm talking about is the most advertised junk foods and beverages we all know of.

Addiction means we are in some way dependent, on a substance and don't think we can go without it.

When a person is, for lack of better term, addicted to S.A.D.C.R.A.P. (especially if they think they can get away with making progress without interrupting their dependency), everything that comes out of their mouth and every intention is a manipulation to get more of the substance they are emotionally attached to, whether its alcohol or excessive cheese or sugar itself...they are pre-occupied with S.A.D.C.R.A.P. There's simply no rational reasoning or motivating with a person who is in an addictive cycle. Everything that comes out of their mouth is directly or indirectly an attempt to manipulate the situation to get more of what they are dependent on.

Having enough B.N.B.B.s on board directly interferes with addiction through the brain/chemical/emotional connection.

Chapter conclusion:

When you notice yourself reaching for, eyeing or putting S.A.D.C.R.A.P. in your body, it indicates one or more B.N.B.B.s are too low in the brain (for you). The B.N.B.B.s eliminate all kinds of cravings.

"If I turned around and watched him fly away I wouldn't be a be surprised." Y.H., Seattle, WA

Chapter Twenty

The Fitness-lifestyle
Is An Inconvenience To The Fat-lifestyle

The fitness-lifestyle is not just about food.

When you think of any lifestyle whether a musician, a doctor, a realtor or athlete, there are all kinds of things that go with that particular lifestyle.

One of the big surprises to people in the precontemplation and contemplation stages is that the ways they have been living to get fat have to be exchanged for becoming lean and healthy...*permanently!*

Think of a musician without a musical instrument...a realtor without a phone...a doctor without a white coat and stethoscope. Regardless of the focus, you have to get the things, be around the people and develop the habits which support your chosen life goals. If you don't develop the lifestyle itself, then it can be challenging to sustain the drive and look forward to a bright future.

In terms of a fat-loss/fitness-lifestyle it starts with the exercise and nutrition program. You have to have some clothing and shoes conducive to your workouts. You have to figure out what whole-foods, functional-foods and dietary supplements you need. Eventually, you'll begin developing more social connections in addition to the other ones you already have which re-enforces your decision to get healthy once and for all. And you'll see clothing that you'd like to wear during workouts. You might see a fitness tracker or heart rate monitor that will help you track your progress. If you have an old bike you might start looking at new ones and a helmet and cycling shoes.

Although exercise and nutrition consistency is the primary key to your success, the other things support your decision to turn-over-a-new-leaf and *build a fitness-lifestyle for yourself.*

These other things don't seem important in their own right, incidental really, but one commonality I've seen among the people who don't follow through is they don't surrender to the process of a fitness-lifestyle (it conflicts with the self-image of being fat) or they don't believe giving up their fat-lifestyle will be as enjoyable as their fit-lifestyle. Once a person comes to terms with what it takes to really be healthy, they begin accessorizing their selves which shows engagement in the process the same as they were doing accessorizing the fat-lifestyle with spending time, energy and money on S.A.D.C.R.A.P., junk food, coffees, nails, hair, clothes to fit an unfit body and so on.

One of the ways trainers can tell if you're engaged in your own fitness journey is if you're investing the same time, energy and money you were to get fat in the first place, in things that support your fat-loss lifestyle. If you aren't, then it hints to a lack of commitment and a possible belief that the changes are short-term rather than a lifestyle change...that fat-loss happens "to you" versus something you're engaged in like buying a cup of coffee.

I have an Army buddy (Rob) who started a fat-loss program six weeks ago from the time I'm writing this sentence. He decided to use cycling as his cardiovascular training and had an initial goal of about 50-60 pounds of fat he wanted to lose. He started posting on Facebook right away about his intentions (excitement). He told how his Army buddy is helping with his nutrition program. He showed pictures of his bike (equipment). He showed maps of his bike routes he was taking with a GPS tracker that shows duration, mileage, time, etc. (enthusiasm). Rob asked me about a body composition testing scale. I texted him the link to Amazon and he went right on to purchase it without hesitation before we were done talking (he wants to know his progress for sure). He showed other bike helmets and shoes he is considering and gives reviews of the equipment he is using (paying it forward). Rob referred others to me and continues posting how he got all his questions answered to make his progress easier and more effective. Even in the rain he says, *"It's a good day to ride."* (positive attitude and lack of excuses). In about six weeks he has lost 24 pounds, so far (I consider 12-20 pounds per month as a measure of effectiveness).

The point being that Rob has built a fitness-lifestyle and is building up his surrounding and looking at ways to be more accountable through technology. He's excited and taking action without trying to argue or negotiate his way out of doing the work to reach is goals. Rob takes responsibility to maintain the emotional state required to succeed.

He says, *"Thanks man, feeling so much better...it's crazy how much the mental side plays...you have to retrain your mind too..it's all about self control when eating and making the right choices."*

This is a great example of the type of clients who make the industry especially enjoyable.

Chapter conclusion:

Build your life and surroundings up to support your goals.

"Sovereign, Thank you for your time and sharing your knowledge with our future leaders. The feedback was very positive and helps to better emphasize the importance of what we seem to be harping on them about."

Thanks again,

Paul Fowler, CPT Assistant Professor of Military Science

MSU Billings, MT

Chapter Twenty-One

Separate Emotions From The Actions

One of the easier ways to talk about the dynamic(s), that people who are successful with their fat-loss program exhibit, it is that even though they are having emotions and often strong emotions, they simply get in, do their work out and nutrition, but set their feelings "aside" in order to exercise and get enough nutrition, just like Rob does.

This is not to say that emotions are not important, significant or essential...they are all that and more! It's just that people who are successful in any category are able to feel their feelings, but keep moving forward...keep moving forward...stay engaged in the doing.

Any strategy you utilize or create, as long as you acknowledge you're having a feeling, name the feeling you're experiencing and then set it aside or even release it for the time will likely be effective.

How to know if your strategy is working or not comes down to one question: *"Are you doing your exercise and nutrition!?"* Proper nutrition is 80% of the success you get or miss out on!

I've had clients who know what the B.N.B.B.s mean and skip them then constantly ask me about other products that are known to be inert or even dangerous. They skip the fundamentals, but want to add other stuff that is a waste of time, energy and money. If you don't trust your trainer's suggestions, (or refuse to follow them), then you should look for a different trainer. If you don't put what your trainer suggests to use, then you don't develop a standard of instincts. Instincts come from doing correct actions, but if you skip steps that your trainer says to do, you're unwittingly holding out on yourself! As a trainer, I'll work with somebody for one cycle to give them time to get it together, but after that if they continue to skip my suggestions, I refer them on. They have to be congruently ready and be in a state of mind of, *"Show and tell me exactly what I have to do to get the results I want."* If they skip stuff, they aren't ready.

I was reading an article by another nationally recognized trainer about a female client who insists she wants to get the same quality results as his other clients but won't even take a single protein supplement, then complains she isn't getting fast enough results.

This is what anyone in any category of success will tell you they do...feel it and move forward anyway. If you don't think you'll be able to exercise or as though you're paralyzed by the feelings that are coming up, there's two things happening: 1) You're identifying with the feelings more than you are with the goals you'll accomplish and who you'll be at the time of accomplishment and 2) You're letting the feelings take up the space and energy that is required to do your workouts and nutrition.

Some people utilize what is referred to as "sub-modality" work. This consists of giving more sensory attributes to the feeling. For example, *"This feeling is orange (color/visual), its loud (sound/auditory), its rough in texture (kinesthetic/feeling), it smells like apples (olfactory/smell) and tastes like watermelon (taste/gustatory)."*

The point of this exercise is to make conscious a thing that has been having unconscious influence and then adding descriptive details that your conscious mind can work with without having to summon the details/content of the feeling. This exercise can be done in 30 seconds and then you simply set it aside so perceptually it's not inside as much. If it seems like it's still connected, then you can imagine a string connected to you, thank the feelings for all the help it has provided and then set it free by snipping the line in your imagination.

The point is not to discount or dismiss the importance of feelings or emotions, but to begin the process of learning to simply notice, acknowledge, experience and release them so you can move forward with the rest of your future. The whole process can be done silently, to yourself in a minute or less. If nothing else, as feelings come up, simply give them the sub-modality descriptors that match your experience and then picture setting them aside for the time.

This exercise will be the beginning of balancing the emotions and demonstrate that you are not your emotions. Emotions enhance life experience and with people who haven't made the distinction between their identity and what they are feeling, this exercise helps distinguish the physical & mental you from transient feelings that have historically been contained and prevented from moving on and making way for what's yet to come.

If this exercise isn't an exact match, then be creative and come up with your own model. As long as you are noticing, then acknowledging, then naming and setting aside/releasing the emotions (and maybe even thanking them for the help they have provided), you'll likely be on track in this sense.

The next phase of the process has to do with if you keep having the same memories, resentments, recall of hurts (incidents or people who you perceive hurt you), traumas, etc., coming into mind. If this is the case for you (it happens to everyone) then this most likely indicates that forgiveness needs to happen to permanently free you from your past.

You can utilize just about any kind of strategy that separates emotions that are inhibiting your actions and to gain control of emotions, rather than being controlled by your emotions. If in doubt, ask for help!

A positive-assertive attitude is what Rob exhibits in his fitness-lifestyle. He is positive (versus pessimistic or negative), assertive (meaning he goes after it rather than behaving like he's waiting for it to "happen to him") and maintains his attitude. Rob takes what I tell him to do, does it as I instructed him to do including rest days and nutritional components and doesn't change anything or skip anything. If in doubt, he texts me from his home or job in a couple states away to give updates (proactive) and ask questions (engaged).

One of the most common strategies successful people use to maintain their attitude is calling up pleasant memories to build a platform of emotional stability. Even if they don't feel like doing something in the moment, they go about creating the emotional state that supports the goal at hand and then do behaviors that match the current goals. *Imagine your success and feel that now.* One of the productive uses of emotions is to re-enforce the behaviors you want more of...by recalling the positive emotions you are doing the first step to laying down habits of continued successful actions.

A common stumbling block is when someone's self-image is a match for what the [past] has been like versus what they want their future to be like. One of the most successful factors for making your habits easier is to create an image in your mind of how you want to become and then summon the emotions to match that image. As your image improves or updates, the behaviors, your self talk, gut-feelings, intuition and habits will align more with where you are headed rather than where you have been.

By asking yourself, *"What came before this?"* you'll begin developing conscious continuity of cause-and-effect and notice how much control you actually have over your level of body-fat separate from the emotions.

Self *dis*-esteem refers to when we do things that seem to feel good in the moment but are detrimental to healthy self-esteem in the long run. These behaviors lower a person's self-esteem and ironically, the more they do behaviors and make poor choices which erode the self-esteem the more they do behaviors that erode self-esteem. At some point you have to simply force yourself (overcome inertia) to do behaviors that build your self-esteem and health. From there you continue on with the process. Success breeds success.

When you feel impulsive or compulsive, meaning you think you might want to buy some S.A.D.C.R.A.P. even though it's not in alignment with your goals, it points to a habit that is charged with the emotions of anxiety...like you can't stop yourself. As you delay your response and examine, *"What came before this?"* you'll gain insight to the emotional drivers and motivations making a previous unconscious process conscious. You get to decide whether you'll charge productive habits in alignment with your goals or destructive habits which derail your intentions. If you tend to be anxious and it interferes, work to turn the anxiousness into excitement for your workout. You can do that!

As you gain confidence and competence you'll find you can rise above the emotional states that previously side-tracked, distracted and derailed you. By doing so, you'll likely gain side benefits like self-confidence, courage, and faith that your goal is already been attained.

Chapter conclusion:

By separating the emotions that interfere with your actions and replacing them with emotions which produce motivation and drive, you're laying the groundwork for habits which make you feel more comfortable when you're doing them then when you're not.

"I am already getting more strength and definition than I have ever had and it's only been four workouts!...people are commenting that I look different already!!" B.R., Seattle, WA

Chapter Twenty-Two

A Simple, But Very Effective
Model For Freeing Yourself From Pain

Now, I'll give you a heads-up right from the get-go that this is not a book on religion. Although I was raised going to church, in my experience people find the spiritual model that is right for them at the time that is appropriate for them. I have my own experiences, but I don't try to convince others to go to church or anything along those lines. I don't convince people to pursue any particular model. And I usually don't share this kind of information with people unless I know them pretty well (people don't want to hear it)...*owning and identifying with pain.*

I have found that some of the principles that were taught when I was a little kid going to Sunday School, tended to come back around for me as an adult, but not really the way I thought they were taught.

One of the most difficult and challenging practices...but most rewarding in terms of return-on-investment, is learning what I refer to as forgiveness. I know, I know a touchy subject. If you have already realized this then you're ahead of the game.

What I'm about to show you is my best interpretation of a process I have used extensively and successfully. Everyone I have shown this to has had equally measurable results. I think it's really amazing, but I didn't invent it, I simply am describing what has been taught for thousands of years, at least.

In my experiences, the first 15 years of my life were the most challenging in the sense that the quantity, quality, intensity and frequency of stress was so much that it was difficult to sort out. Before one stress was done the next one was happening. I'm one of those people who when people know what my life was like they can't believe I turned out how I did or that I even made it, without destroying myself. Then adult life kicked in which was essentially recovery time from those years, but that's when, for lack of better terms, I didn't have much in the way of healthy coping skills. I simply did the best I could and kept focused on the future. All along the way, as I pointed out earlier, I observed and paid attention to everyone all along the way, essentially learning vicariously from others. In hindsight, I can see where all those challenges and stressors were simply preparing me and temporing me for what was ahead.

Long story short, when we get hurt, in any way, a lot of people tuck the hurt away like a mental note so to protect the self and not let it happen the same way again. Sometimes we don't have control over the situation and we don't have a way to prevent things from happening again. The short part of the story is that people tend to harbor anger, resentment and hold others accountable in our minds/hearts. Sometimes the pain of losing people is the least of the pain had they stayed around.

Harboring resentment kinda, sorta works in the short run since you have to adapt and get stronger and more resilient in the moment, but like the stress hormones (adrenaline and cortisol), they work good in the short-term for quick healing, but if they go on, as in chronic stress they break the body down.

A lot of what is keeping people from getting the goals they want is being emotionally stuck in the past. What's often keeping people stuck in the past is anger and resentment for things that happen and ways others hurt them. For lack of better ways to describe this, pain causes people to attempt to [control] in order to prevent hurts from happening again, whether physical, mental, emotional or spiritual. Sometimes you'll hear people talking about holding people who hurt them accountable, which in itself is control over the past.

The Catch-22 is that the more a person tries to control others, or the past or even justifies their anger toward people or situations, the less control they tend to have over themselves. You simply can't control others without it having some reciprocal affect on yourself. But the crux of it is that the more resentment or anger you hold, the more it hurts you. It's simply non-negotiable. But in reality, holding images, feelings, thoughts and memories about past hurts is that like suppressing emotions in general, the longer they are held the more and more energy it takes to keep them held.

From a strictly healing/holisitic standpoint, it comes down to the fact that we "get" a certain amount of energy each day and part of what that energy is used for is to heal the physical, mental, emotional and spiritual aspects of our beings...*kind of an energy-savings account.* The energy used to suppress emotions and hold resentment and anger taps into or makes withdrawls from the energy savings account that is prioritized for health and fitness, but doesn't give us a health return...in fact it has the opposite effect.

People can increase the amount of this energy and expand on its positive effects on the health, but not as long as energy is being squandered on anger and resentment or holding others accountable in their mind...*nature simply doesn't work that way.*

Again, this is the best way I can describe this, but considering I began my career as a licensed massage practitioner, got certified in reflexology, Reiki and a ton of other hands-on, healing modalities, this is the best I can do. What I can tell you is that if you do that kind of work and you're paying attention at all, you notice where the mind, emotions and energy merge with and affect physical health and energy. I can't say I have the market on how to describe the process, but I can certainly provide you with a model that doesn't contradict any spiritual model I know of. And the best part is that you don't have to take my word for it. You can experiment with it in an honest and intentional way and find out for yourself. I think you'll be amazed, even if its review for you.

Forgiveness:

I was one of the most skeptical people of models of forgiveness. I couldn't figure out how things I thought or remembered could be affecting my physical world or my goals or physical health. But I've found many categories over the decades where you could say mind and matter merge, or where spirit and physical affect each other directly. Energy and information is the basis of everything known.

In relation to the emotions of fat-loss, how this ties in is that your body and mind tell you where you need to start to clean up the past and move on. It's so simple. If you think of a person or place or situation that you consider a painful experience, that's where you start...it's that simple.

The body has innate knowledge of itself and if you pay attention to it, it will tell you step by step, in sequence which thing is the next to be cleaned up (resolved) for you to reach your goals be they physical, mental, emotional or spiritual. Those four categories are all tied into one another and are used as needed depending on the situation. But, when out of balance, they affect each other equally too.

When you have cleared an incident up (fully forgiven and released it), your body will tell you the next one because it will pop into your mind. The process continues. Sometimes, one incident will keep coming up. This indicates more emphasis/intention needs to be on step one. If it's about a person that is related to repeated incidents, by the same person(s), then do the process for each incident. If you aren't clearly intent on letting the person or memory go, the positive effects will be limited. Forgiveness works because it enables you to release control of the past, thereby freeing up your energy in the present.

So, pick the first thing that comes to mind. It doesn't matter what it is, since your body will tell you which one matters to it the most right now in this moment. I could pick being punched in the face or having something stolen or being betrayed, it doesn't matter. The point is to learn the system.

First Step: *"I forgive (name of person) for such and such...."*

(This releases the person from affecting your energy or being an energy draw, directly or indirectly anymore). If it helps, picture them being released.

Step Two: *"I forgive myself for my participation or naivety in the situation of..."*

(Accidentally holding unconscious resentment toward the self for either not knowing better, letting the self down or for unwittingly participating releases another energy drain). Even if you know you had nothing to do with it or any control over the situation, do this step anyway, you'll realize why later, after you've become proficient.

Step Three: *"I ask for forgiveness, from..."*

(Whatever your model of spirituality is, apply it here.) This applies to the concept of a higher power, and even if it doesn't make sense, do it anyway. In other words, if you believe in God, *"I ask God for forgiveness for my participation in such and such..."* If you have a different belief system, apply that here.

It also applies to faith, that everything is going to be ok.

Step Four: Say anything you're grateful for, regardless how trivial. Like a lot of other exercises herein, the content/details don't matter...the important part is in the habit or context/big picture of doing it.

If you're so down that you honestly don't feel grateful for anything, say you're grateful for something insignificant, like the dirt or grass: *"I'm thankful for the grass"*.

Sounds crazy I know, but what these five steps do is realign how you're using energy and it doesn't matter if you're thankful, as long as you do the exercise. Just like you don't get fit from the first day you exercise, it's the *process* that works *cumulatively*, not the first exercise or multivitamin you take.

By saying you're thankful for something that doesn't seem relevant to you, the emotional and energetic content begins to realign to a healthy state. By doing this, you'll start noticing things you truly are grateful for, which begins releasing you from your past and aligning you with the present...you'll begin noticing a free-feeling, a sense of lightness, like a weight has been lifted. This begins the process of bridging you to your goals that have seemed out of reach and connects you to the goals you see and experience as accomplished in your future.

There's nothing magical or mysterious about this, it's just the proper use of energy, will, intention and a lot of people haven't learned about it...*that's how they get emotionally stuck...accidently.*

Step Five/Final Step: Say something you're looking forward to: *"I'm looking forward to burning fat and being fit once and for all."*

You can say whatever you want. You can do this whenever you want. I personally like doing it when I wake up and right before going to sleep, but any time a memory or a pain comes up, simply work through it.

The biggest roadblock to people doing this simple practice is when they are addicted to the negativity and control, itself. Negativity is familiar and comforting, at first. They haven't turned it over, lack faith that everything will be ok if they let it go. To some people, who haven't experienced how good it feels to let go the people who hurt you go, they perceive the peak control experience as holding resentment (energetic prisoner)..e.g. *"If no one else can hold the bad person accountable, I certainly will."* But you can't hold another accountable without holding yourself accountable...*it just doesn't work that way.*

Holding people or situations accountable (even if they are difficult to comprehend or understand) uses energy of the person doing the holding that they could have used for their own health and well-being...*its depleting.* Resentment, control and anger feel good at first, but ultimately, people become kind of enslaved (lack of better term) by the negativity...when they insist they are "right" for holding resentment or holding someone accountable, they get a psychological "high" and then perceive that letting go the feeling of being in control might make them vulnerable. Most people don't enjoy being hurt or betrayed! That's normal. But when preventing being hurt has a boomerang affect on the self and they don't know it, they have essentially moved from the victim role to the violator role, insisting who hurt them but actually hurting themselves, through misuse of personal energy/power.

I have seen that people don't really get away with hurting others...it always comes around.

In short, resentment and anger causes pain (physical, mental, emotional & spiritual) through exhaustion of the mind and body, via adrenaline and cortisol hormone systems. When people hold resentment and anger the side effects are that the stress hormones are triggered long after the incident is done and gone. The stress hormones exhaust the body and mind outside awareness.

The bright side is that the process reverses, pretty readily, once the five-step process is applied whole heartily and thoroughly.

Chapter conclusion:

Developing the habit of forgiveness will likely provide you energy you have been wondering why you didn't have.

Any place where you are giving away emotional energy without a positive return, will leave you in a negative energy deficit, thereby creating fatigue and depression. Negativity, negative-visualization, recycling the past and co-dependency, as well as holding grudges, refusing to forgive-and-forget and live in gratitude are key players in this category.

"My workouts are better because of what he taught me. What I like most about training with Sovereign is the information and his honesty." J.G., First Hill, Seattle

Chapter Twenty-Three

How To Get More Of What
You Want, *But Don't/Haven't Had So Far*

Gratitude is a thing I describe and experience as a process-phenomena, which enables people to get what they want most, whether stated to others or not and which brings more of which you are grateful for, even if you haven't had it before.

The idea of gratitude can be bridged between religious or spiritual teachings & mind over matter teachings. On one hand, everything is available or possible and on another-hand, there's the concept of the late Napoleon Hill said: *"Whatever your mind can conceive and believe the mind can achieve, regardless of how many times you may have failed in the past."*

What I have found is that (and no, I'm not going to take the position of proving it to the "negative-nannies" but you can prove or disprove it to yourself) you can get, receive, experience and become whatever you want, but if you want to keep it, the thing can't hurt or take away from another person. In other words, you can override balance and get a thing at-any-cost, but to keep the thing or not have a negative rebound effect, it cannot initially hurt or take away from others and yes, you can use whatever abundance you receive to at least in part help improve others with it, even if only to help others do the same. With that in mind, we know that not everyone who complains wants a solution. Many people complain simply to unnaturally gain sympathy and energy from others around them, rather than gaining energy naturally through accomplishment and natural means, but I digress.

One of (if not THE) reasons which inhibit people getting what they want is purely perceptual...perceiving that it's in the future or 'away' from you keeps 'pushing' the thing or the experience into the future in a kind of unconscious procrastination.

The idea of identity ties into this... in other words, a person will never sustain a thing if it conflicts with their unconscious (out of awareness) self-image (how they see themselves in the world). Everything is available, even to the point of defying rationale and logic and scientific proof. The mind is designed by function to prove you are right (reticular-activating system), so whatever you intend to be right about, the mind will go about pulling evidence from your environment whether you insist a thing is true or not, your mind will gather the information to prove it! That's partly why two different people, even twins, can be in the same place but have a different experience, memory and perception of it. And that's a reason why people who obsess and can't break free from certain thoughts seem to get locked into circular-logic. The good news is that you can start fresh and reinvent yourself-image at any time...it's not left to chance. *Psychocybernetics* by Maxwell Maltz goes into great detail about this.

A seeming limit to this at this time is that we can't bring people back from death since that is related to affecting control over another or another's higher purpose, but the idea of wanting to points to unresolved pain and grief. In this case, the balanced choice is to gain relief of the pain of loss & grief versus trying to bring someone back from the dead, beyond medical and life saving endeavors.

So, the practice of gratitude simply means that instead of wishing, hoping, and putting off, you connect the desire of what you want with the emotions of having already completing or accomplishing or receiving the thing and make it in your mind as though the thing has already happened, even if it means recycling positive memories of previous accomplishments in the new context to "charge" the accomplishment. Then watch it come to pass. It's the mental and emotional behavior of behaving/feeling "as if" that frees you up from the mental processes and idiosyncrasies that would otherwise interfere with the accomplishment outside conscious awareness...*also known as faith.*

Here's how it breaks down:

1) Be clear what you want without conflicting interests 2) Combine with the emotions of anticipation, excitement and accomplishment that you got what you wanted 3) Create the feelings that

you just received it and all that goes with it 4) Say and feel how grateful you are that it came to pass 5) Repeat the process 6) For added kick, invest some time adding the feeling of fear to the mix (fear charges and attracts the thing we're fearful of, even when it's something you really want).

What you're effectively doing is updating yourself-image of who you are in the world, which changes what things your mind filters/directs your brain to pay attention to (reticular activating system), so you in turn notice things that were there all along, but seem to appear out of nowhere (noticed opportunity).

The size of the thing is irrelevant, unless you convince yourself that the magnitude is relevant. If you tend to need evidence before you can believe it, then start with small seemingly insignificant things that you aren't as attached to so that it doesn't conflict with your beliefs. If you lack faith, then cultivate your faith first.

If you want the big thing right off and you believe you can do it, then it just comes down to allowing your mental walls of what you perceive as possible to dissolve away and then really, really put the majority of your energy in this to feeling grateful of the thing having come to pass (faith). The speed of the thing coming to pass is in relation to you getting the part of your mind out of the way that would normally not believe it until you see it, enough to let the thing come into your life.

The mistake that most make is thinking they have to receive before they can have faith and feel grateful...that's backwards.

Remember, whatever proof you want and pay attention to, so shall you get. That means if you'd rather be right than have what you say you want, you'll be right but not get what you want.

[Change occurs in an instant], but for most people they believe "this and that" has to occur first, which is them interfering in the things they insist they want! In other words, they develop rules that they live by, but the rules aren't necessarily real to everyone, they were created like a superstition. If two people come together this way for the same outcome, the result can be more dynamic, but no one is limited except by the rules they make up to live by, in their mind (superstition). Enjoy the process!

Chapter conclusion:

Practice being grateful for what you want, as though you already have, have become or are living what you want before you have evidence its real. Pay attention to what happens.

"I did the nutrition stuff you showed me … it had an extraordinary affect." R.P., Billings, MT

Chapter Twenty-Four

You Have To Do It For Yourself

Healthy, sustainable fat-loss is something you engage in and do for yourself. No one can do it [to you] nor [for you] no matter how much you pay them. If you're burning less than 12-20 pounds of fat per month, either the program isn't designed correctly for fat-loss or you are something is getting inadvertently changed that is critical to success, thinking you're doing it correctly, but not. Or you're skipping key parts that cannot be skipped. There's no mysteries to healthy fat-loss anymore.

"...you have helped me more than you know." S.L., Seattle, WA

Pre-training Questionnaire:

Have you had professional nutrition training before?

___Yes ___No

Are you coachable and open to whole-foods nutrition suggestions?

___Yes ___No

Would you follow through on my suggestions?   ___Yes ___No

Did you know that your fitness/fat-loss success or lack thereof is about 80%, based on the how well you apply the three parts of nutrition, during/from the first month, of your program?

___Yes ___No

Have you had professional B.N.B.B.s training?

___Yes ___No

Are you coachable and open to suggestions about which B.N.B.B.s to take, for optimal results? (versus picking a program apart).

___Yes ___No

Currently participating in a structured, resistance-training?

___Yes ___No

If so, frequency/duration of sessions ?_________________________________.

Have you had professional personal training before?

___Yes ___No

Have you had fat-burning cardio-respiratory training before?

___Yes ___No

Is it realistic for you to prioritize 3-4 hours each week to exercise?

___Yes ___No

What is your current bodyfat percentage?_____________________________.

How much fat do you want to lose?_________________________________.

What has been your biggest challenge(s), in regard to fat-loss?

____.

Pre-training Questionnaire continued:

Are you committed to applying yourself to resistance-training, cardiovascular-training, and the 3 parts of nutrition: (1) Whole-foods, 2) Functional-foods, & 3) The B.N.B.B.s *for at least one year?* (versus a person who starts stuff, but doesn't follow through).

___Yes ___No

With a standard of 12-20 pounds per month, how long could it take you to lose that amount of fat?_______________________________.

How many different weight loss programs have you tried, before?

____.

I look for people who have tried a few things that didn't work and who are looking for something that definetely works. Are you the type of person who wants a structured program that tells you exactly what to do throughout the day, so nothing is left to chance?

___Yes ___No

Are you willing to get your B.N.B.B.s squared away from the beginning of your program?

___Yes ___No

Although you will likely begin to see and feel positive improvements right away, peramanent fat-loss requires a lifestyle change. Are you willing to become more fit, by taking one day at a time, committing to a program that definitely works, for at least one year,?

___Yes ___No

How long have you been wanting to lose weight?_________________.

Imagine you have lost all the fat you ever wanted to, have more energy and look better then ever and all that is taken care of. In what way(s) would your life improve, as a result?

____.

*You may find it helpful to remove these pages, scan them and email them to me to assist with your complimentary consulatation.

Afterword

As a licensed health care provider, author, speaker and fitness professional I know from my own experiences what it feels like to want to improve my health, do what I think is right and still not get the kind of results I expected. I am sure you have your own goals and are looking forward to achieving them. I believe you are capable of living the life of your dreams in your healthy, ideal-self body and you will achieve your dreams.

By learning about how emotions fuel your goals and how your body utilizes the B.N.B.B.s you can have more control over your life and get what you want for less time, energy and money. You can prevent many of the most common *dis*-eases of today and burn fat faster than you have before.

I want you to contact me today and tell me about all the positive benefits you have experienced, as a result of this information!

In my experience, the greatest potential problem is in not educating yourself about it, but in simply doing it.

I cannot wait to hear from you. I especially cannot wait to share your success story with others.

Appendix

For your complimentary consultation, contact the author at the email below or through Facebook Messenger at Sov Valentine:

e-mail:

sovereignmv@gmail.com

My website:

http://sovereign-valentine.mykajabi.com

Sovereign Valentine
CFT, CET, Yft, SSC, SPN, Cft, GFI, SFI, CERT, CMCht, Reiki Master

Reasons or Results! Training Systems© 2018